REPETITIVE STRAIN INJURY

REPETITIVE STRAIN INJURY
A Computer User's Guide

EMIL PASCARELLI, M.D. • DEBORAH QUILTER

Foreword by Fred Hochberg, M.D.
Director, Musical Medicine Clinic
Massachusetts General Hospital

John Wiley & Sons, Inc.
New York • Chichester • Brisbane • Toronto • Singapore

Library of Congress Cataloging-in-Publication Data:

Pascarelli, Emil F.
   Repetitive strain injury: a computer user's guide/
Emil Pascarelli, Deborah Quilter.
      p. cm.
   Includes index.
   ISBN 0-471-59532-2 (acid-free paper).—ISBN 0-471-59533-0
(acid-free paper : pbk.)
    1. Overuse injuries. 2. Computer terminals–Health aspects.
I. Quilter, Deborah, 1950– . II. Title.
RD97.6.P37 1994
617.5'7044–dc20   93-31758

Printed in the United States of America.

10 9 8 7 6 5 4 3 2

To D. K. Pascarelli (from EP)

To E. R. P. (from DQ)

Foreword

Repetitive strain injury is hardly a new phenomenon: It was noted among telegraphers and other manual tradesmen as early as the mid-nineteenth century.

Now RSI has hit the largest single occupational group ever—computer users. Studies performed by industry and occupational health physicians reveal that one-fifth to one-quarter of computer keyboard users (both vocational and recreational) have symptoms referable to their activity.

To treat these injuries, doctors have applied old-fashioned methods of treatment: splints, anti-inflammatories, and surgery. However, too little effort has been paid to prevention, which is a surprise considering the staggering costs associated with RSI.

Now, through the efforts of Dr. Emil Pascarelli at the Miller Health Care Institute, considerable light has been cast on the causes and cure of repetitive strain injury. *Repetitive Strain Injury: A Computer User's Guide* represents the first workable solution to RSI, in a comprehensive, concise format. The book tells computer users everything they need to know about RSI, and it should be on the desk of every computer user in America.

Fred Hochberg, M.D.

Preface

Emil Pascarelli, M.D.

My experience with RSI began in 1985, when we opened the Miller Institute for Performing Artists and began to treat injured musicians, many of whom spent long hours preparing for stressful events such as concerts or auditions. Their complaints of pain and weakness involved the upper body, hands, forearms, and shoulders. By watching the musicians play their instruments, I realized that most of their woes stemmed from a combination of improper technique, ill-fitting instruments, and poor physical conditioning. To treat this multifaceted problem, I prescribed retraining so the musicians could learn to play without doing further damage, and rehabilitation to improve their posture and overall fitness level.

Shortly thereafter, computer users with similar symptoms started appearing at the Miller Institute, only many of them were much more severely injured than the musicians. Again, when I watched them type, I realized that the same culprits that plagued the musicians bedeviled the computer operators—improper technique, poor fit between human and instrument, and lack of physical conditioning and postural awareness. By applying methods similar to those we used with the musicians, we were able to help many of them, too.

Almost a decade ago, few people had heard of RSI. Today, public consciousness of this problem has grown. However, misconceptions about RSI abound and RSI is the source of much confusion and controversy among medical professionals, some of whom still think that many of the symptoms are simply a manifestation of the normal aches and pains we all experience from time to time. After examining over a thousand patients, many of whose careers were threatened and sometimes ended by RSI, it seemed obvious that this was a serious and growing occupational health problem and not just "aches and pains."

To add to the confusion, many people who complained of wrist pain were diagnosed as having carpal tunnel syndrome without the variety of other problems they had being taken into consideration. Carpal tunnel syndrome became almost synonymous with RSI, and this development appears to have diverted many clinician's attention from a broader view of the problem.

I am often asked why this did not happen to people who worked on typewriters. In the early days of the typewriter, hitting the keys too rapidly would jam the typebars. The QWERTY keyboard was introduced by the Remington

Arms Company in 1873 to distribute the workload throughout the keyboard and avoid jamming. Over time, productivity increased with improvements in the mechanical typewriter. The typewriter allowed built-in rest time for the correction of errors and the insertion of paper. Because the keys were stepped, people supported their arms and wrists with their upper body. With the advent of the flat keyboard, this all changed. The new keyboard looked innocent enough, except that now people could rest their hands on the desk to use the keys. It could handle all you could type at any speed, even beyond human capability, yet because there was no paper involved, errors were corrected with additional keystrokes and rest breaks were taken less frequently. Bent wrists, contorted postures, and strained forearms and hands became far more common. As more people used computers, the incidence of RSI increased; in the 1990s, injury and disability have reached epidemic proportions. Over the years, our work has shown us that the causes of RSI are multiple, and a treatment plan needs to address them all in a coordinated way. This book attempts to make that point clear.

The person who deserves much of the credit for this book is my coauthor, Deborah Quilter, a talented journalist who became a victim of RSI. She proposed that we write this book together and I happily agreed. Much of the material in this book is the result of the endless hours she spent researching the literature and listening to patients. Most importantly, because of the broad knowledge she gained in over two years of intensive work coupled with her own bout with RSI, she has contributed many original, unique, and useful concepts to assist computer users. The result of our work together is a book created to help those already dealing with RSI and to prevent others from developing it. We hope you, the reader, find this information useful.

Preface

Deborah Quilter

I was diagnosed with repetitive strain injury in 1991. If I knew then what I know now, it never would have happened.

Like many people, I had symptoms for at least a year before I sought treatment. Then one night I had a scary experience. I had been putting in long hours (50 to 60 hours a week, sometimes 16 hours a day). But after working late this particular night, about 4:00 A.M. I noticed that my arms were so heavy and tired I could hardly hold them to the keyboard. Odd, I thought: Wasn't I accustomed to these hours? A strange electrical charge buzzed through my gut. Something was wrong.

At the time, RSI wasn't front-page news, and when the press did cover it, repetitive strain injury was invariably equated with carpal tunnel syndrome. The stories usually described an affliction that seemed to be computer-related, but they didn't say what you could do to prevent it, other than swearing off computers completely. The reports generally focused on one symptom, wrist pain, which wasn't a problem for me. My forearms felt like they were on fire, though—a common symptom of RSI—but the articles didn't mention that. Besides, my symptoms came and went, so I shrugged them off.

Then I read a newspaper account of a woman with such bad computer-related RSI that she could not dress her infant. This piece of information sent chills down my spine. None of the other news stories said RSI could be permanently debilitating! I vowed to get a diagnosis, but I didn't know any doctors who specialized in the hand. Fortunately, I remembered writing an article a few years earlier about the Miller Institute for Performing Artists at St. Luke's/Roosevelt Hospital, founded by Dr. Emil Pascarelli. I liked Dr. Pascarelli's philosophy: namely, to keep performers working by showing them how to prevent injuries through safe technique. Because I feared that any other doctor might tell me to stop writing, I made an appointment with Dr. Pascarelli.

Hundreds of other injured computer users had preceded me to his "performance evaluation" room, and much to my delight, Dr. Pascarelli asked informed questions about my workstation, hours, and computer keyboard. He even had a simulated workstation set up in his office. He videotaped me typing, pointed out the injurious habit that had caused most of my grief (I held up my pinkie when I typed), and showed me how to work without strain. Dr. Pascarelli diagnosed forearm tendinitis and prescribed physical therapy and technique retraining, and the road to recovery began.

When I compared notes with injured friends, I was puzzled. *They* didn't have their muscles carefully tested for an hour and a half by their doctors. *They* weren't videotaped at a simulated workstation. *They* weren't getting technique retraining. Their doctors were seeing them for ten minutes and giving them the standard treatment—EMGs, splints, and anti-inflammatories. They didn't seem to be getting better. I was.

By then I realized that because most people who used computers—which includes a large portion of the work force—unwittingly employed dangerous technique, RSI was going to become a major epidemic. Dr. Pascarelli's approach to RSI seemed like the most logical way to combat RSI because it addressed the root of the problem.

There had to be a book. So I said, "Dr. Pascarelli, let's write a book together." He agreed. For the next several months, I interviewed RSI patients.

I could identify with them. When they winced in pain, I sympathized; when they massaged their sore spots, my sore spots would hurt. When they wondered aloud if they would be permanently disabled, I remembered asking myself the same question. I understood their anxiety as I watched them nervously awaiting their appointments in the waiting room.

There were good times, too: the moment of joy when the patients finally understood the source of their problems and their sense of determination to get better. It was reassuring to see that for most of them, that attitude paid off.

During my recovery, people posed the usual questions about RSI to me, too. "Your arm *still* hurts? Well, how come it's not getting better?" People seemed indignant that this treatment didn't seem to be working more quickly. I made the usual mistakes, too. When I felt better, I plunged ahead like a racehorse, only to backslide in recovery. Every relapse would dishearten me: Maybe I wasn't going to get better after all. Maybe my forearm would be sore and fragile for the rest of my life. Maybe all this pacing stuff didn't work.

Then little things began to change: My hands weren't sore in the morning when I woke up. Little by little, I could face doors without dread, because it didn't hurt to open them. Today, I can use my hands almost normally. Almost, because I have learned to be careful with them—something I never thought about before my injury.

Having seen how serious RSI can be, I realized just how lucky I was to escape permanent disability—and wanted to do something to help prevent other people from having to go through the arduous process of recovery. If you have RSI, I hope this book will help guide you through recovery. If you don't have RSI, I hope it will help you prevent injury.

Acknowledgments

Too many friends, colleagues, and acquaintances shared their experience, expertise, and wisdom with us to name them all here, but we want to acknowledge some of the people whose thoughts and experiences so enriched our book.

Jane Bear-Lehman shared a wealth of information about pacing, work tolerance, the activities of daily living, and many other aspects of RSI gained from years of teaching and clinical experience.

George Piligian helped us clarify and embellish many of our thoughts.

Robert Rosenthal, who advised on the psychology of RSI and chronic pain, always seemed to have an answer for the thorniest life questions.

Robert E. Markison, who embodies some of the best qualities of a good surgeon and doctor, prudence and curiosity, shared his knowledge and deep appreciation of the human hand.

Leslie Mullady and Vincent Rossillo generously advised on legal issues.

P J Dempsey, our editor at John Wiley & Sons, wins top marks for having the good judgment to believe in this book.

Narda Lebo, who illustrated the text, brought motion and life to the flat, still page, perfectly conveying the notion that good posture is dynamic, not rigid.

Jacqueline Padovano always managed to dovetail the authors' hectic schedules with unfailing efficiency and good humor.

The entire staff of the Miller Institute should be commended for giving patients high-quality care. However, two members of the rehabilitation therapy staff stand out: Michele Semler and Ellen Kolber, who unselfishly shared valuable professional observations and suggestions for the book. As Deborah Quilter's personal physical therapist, Michele demonstrated the near-miraculous results that this healing art can achieve—even under deadline pressure. John Kella was always warmly supportive and enthusiastic. Katy Keller and Julie Corbett cleverly alliterated the basic elements of good rehabilitation therapy with the initial P for easy recall.

We thank the librarians at the New York Public Library, the medical library at St. Luke's–Roosevelt Hospital, the New York Academy of Medicine, and the Osler Library of the History of Medicine at McGill University in Canada for their help.

Other people who offered valuable observations and suggestions were Sidney Blair, Joseph DePietro, Richard L. Gross, John Haskell, Susan Nobel of the Mount Sinai–Irving J. Selikoff Occupational Health Clinical Center, Ellen R. Peyser, George Satran, Melvin Schrier, James Sheedy, David Sternman, and Clark Taylor.

We are also indebted to our friends and families for their encouragement and support, especially those who sent us newspaper clippings and videotapes and kept us apprised of events outside the New York area: Sheila Quilter Wheeler, Janice Tong, Dolores Pascarelli, Eric Pascarelli, and Chris Quilter.

Most of all, we wish to thank people who must remain nameless, but upon whose histories, experiences, and insights this work is based—the RSI patients themselves. They were a constant source of courage and inspiration for us, and we are most grateful to them all.

Contents

Throughout the text we emphasize the need to consult with doctors for a proper diagnosis and treatment of RSI. This is an extra reminder that no medication, exercise, physical therapy, or other treatment for RSI should be taken or undertaken without consulting a doctor or other qualified professional.

Many people with RSI were interviewed for this book. Their names and other details have been changed to protect their privacy.

PART I

WHAT YOU SHOULD KNOW ABOUT RSI

CHAPTER 1

RSI: A Preventable Tragedy

No sort of exercise is so healthful or harmless that it does not cause serious disorders, that is, when overdone.

— Bernardino Ramazzini, *Disease of Workers,* 1713

In 1981, when IBM proudly unveiled its first personal computer, America fell in love with it in a way reminiscent of an 18-year-old's infatuation with his first sports car. People loved the computer's speed and responsiveness to touch and the mesmerizing colors of its monitor. Magical computing commands made a game of composing, seducing the user to spend hours at the keyboard. The flashing cursor urged the user to keep pace with its lively tempo, which could challenge the fastest typist.

The desire to dance the fingers quickly over the keys, trying to outpace the computer's lightning response, proved as irresistible as wanting to floor the gas pedal in a sports car. Like a healthy 18-year-old who imagines himself to be invulnerable, the average computer user is not thinking about the dangers of speed. It never crosses his mind that he could have an accident.

To its users, the computer was a sophisticated toy. To business, it was a boon to efficiency and productivity. Unfortunately, the explosion of computer use created an ominous shadow—a problem so serious that it has been dubbed "the occupational disease of the '90s": repetitive strain injury. A decade after the introduction of the personal computer, RSI has mushroomed into one of the fastest growing—and most worrisome—problems facing American business.

Unlike a car crash, repetitive strain injury doesn't happen instantaneously. It occurs over minutes, months, and years, creeping up on the user insidiously. RSI, if untreated, can cause irrevocable loss of the use of your hands. Even if you retain full use of your hands, you can never work the same way again once you've been seriously injured. Symptoms recur intermittently; the fear of reinjury haunts you. Meatpackers have known about RSI for years, but because it is relatively new to white-collar workers, many people who have RSI don't realize it until they suddenly find themselves dropping things or experiencing too much pain to work. At this point, severe damage has already occurred to nerves, muscles, and connective tissue.

RSI IS SERIOUS, AND HAS SERIOUS REPERCUSSIONS

Doctors have disagreed with each other, and blamed each other for not doing the right thing. My employers don't know what to believe. I feel like my employers have written me off. My doctor told me to hang my job up. That's a huge decision.

— RSI patient

Though RSI starts at the keyboard, it can be better understood by looking at its typical impact on the sufferers' daily lives, namely, what they *can't* do. Many people with RSI complain about having difficulty opening doors, which requires twisting, pushing, or pulling arm movements. They find themselves losing their grip on the newspaper or telephone; doing the dishes is too painful for them; and they cannot even grasp a hairbrush, much less hold their hands to the keyboard. Social situations can present problems, too. Some people are reluctant to shake hands during an introduction for fear of triggering an episode of pain.

Many people face severe financial problems as a result of repetitive strain injury. The degree varies from the annoyance of watching their grocery bill mount every month because it's too hard to lift the large economy size of a product into the shopping cart, to a reduced paycheck because they can't work their accustomed overtime hours, to catastrophe if they are the sole breadwinner and unable to work. Some people face gut-wrenching terror if they are unable to find a different line of work, particularly if they can't use their hands well anymore—for anything.

What Is RSI?

In simple medical terms, repetitive strain injury (RSI) is defined as a cumulative trauma disorder (CTD) stemming from prolonged repetitive, forceful, or awkward hand movements. Add to that the poor posture and positioning of an out-of-shape worker, ill-fitting furniture, a badly designed keyboard, and the pressure of a heavy or fast-paced workload, and the stage is set for serious injury. The result is damage to the muscles, tendons, and nerves of the neck, shoulder, forearm, and hand, which can cause pain, weakness, numbness, or impairment of motor control.

The medical definition doesn't begin to tell the whole story, however. RSI is a national tragedy because it has drastically disrupted the lives and livelihoods of thousands of Americans. This tragedy is compounded by the fact that it is preventable in most cases.

If you are reading this, you probably already know what RSI is, and you don't need a lot of statistics to back up the pain you can feel in your own body. However, in case you need to convince anybody else RSI is a serious public health problem, here are some impressive numbers: According to a cover story in *Information Week* (November 9, 1992), RSI costs businesses $20 *billion* a year. According to the National Council on Compensation Insurance, the average compensation of an RSI victim is $29,000. RSI accounts for 60% of all job-related injuries, according to the Department of Labor. To make matters more frightening, by the year 2000 three-quarters of all jobs will probably require using a computer.

No one can put a price tag on the human cost in terms of shattered careers, financial ruin, or family members who live in the shadow of a disabled, depressed parent or spouse.

Setting the Stage for Injury: the Causes of RSI

Repetition

The activities that cause RSI seem utterly innocuous to most people. What could possibly be harmful about striking a key at the computer? Nothing—unless you do it several thousand times a day.

Fine hand movements, repeated hour after hour, day after day, thousands upon thousands of times, eventually strain the muscles and tendons of the forearms, wrists, and fingers, causing microscopic tears. Injured muscles tend to contract, decreasing the range of motion necessary for stress-free work. The sheaths that cover delicate tendons run out of lubrication because they aren't given time to rest, so tendon and sheath chafe. Now the insulted tissues become painful. In addition, there can be numbness, tingling, or hypersensitivity to touch. Unless this cycle is interrupted, it repeats itself over and over, and a long-term, chronic problem results.

Some corporations spend millions of dollars buying wrist rests and ergonomic chairs in order to stem the rising tide of repetitive strain injury, but this alone can't solve the problem. Repetitive motions cause repetitive strain injury; thus, the companies that are redesigning jobs to have more variety and safety are using a better approach: addressing the source of RSI.

Ignorance

One of the primary causes of RSI is ignorance about how the hand works. Dr. Robert Markison, a San Francisco hand surgeon, finds three major "pockets of ignorance" in this regard: doctors, who get a mere three hours devoted to the upper limb in medical school; industrial designers who should know how the hand works but don't; and an uninformed lay public that knows nothing about the proper use of the hand.

Strained and Constrained Posture

To stay healthy, the body must move in a balanced way that allows full range of motion, but most computer jobs require excessive upper-body immobility, while the tendons and muscles of the forearms, hands, and fingers overwork.

Just sitting at a desk all day is inherently damaging to your muscles and bones because the body was designed to move. As Stewart B. Leavitt points out in "The Healthy Office of the '90s," early humans did not sit for long periods of time; they squatted, knelt, or reclined. Sitting exhausts the body because the back, leg, and trunk muscles must contract constantly to keep the body erect and still. In computer work, the operator must fight gravity constantly just to hold the arms to the keyboard. "Instead of being restful, the sitting position places continuous stresses and strains on one's body.... Just keeping the head vertical is a strenuous act; muscles of the neck and shoulders must work to keep the head at the top of the cervical spine," Leavitt notes. "This is like balancing a heavy bowling ball atop a series of loosely jointed thread spools; a constant series of very small movements—a static workload—is required to maintain equilibrium. One need only observe an infant learning to sit up to be reminded of the complexities and stresses of the simple act of sitting erect."

To make matters worse, most office furniture does not fit the worker. The chairs in many offices were designed to fit men but are frequently occupied by women. Because women are generally smaller, they must compromise their posture and strain their muscles to work. Conversely, tall or big people feel cramped by their workstations. Yet employers unwittingly treat people as though they all had the same bodies by choosing one-size-fits-all furniture. Most of my patients bitterly bemoan the equipment they must use: They can't lower their tables, and their chairs are often either broken or uncomfortable. But even the best chair won't help if other problems are present. One woman complained that her company had provided everybody with great chairs that had "sixteen pumps and an instruction manual," but not enough people to do the work.

Holding Still

The human body must move to remain in optimum health, but the computer virtually encases people in an invisible straitjacket. Holding muscles still for long periods of time ("static loading") causes discomfort and fatigue. The unvarying rigidity of sitting with the arms extended, staring straight ahead for hours on end, exhausts the body. This is why people who don't type a lot, but sit and stare at a computer screen with hands poised over the keyboard, can be at risk for RSI.

A Deconditioned Workforce

In medicine, if someone is referred to as "deconditioned," it means that the person is out of shape. Most Americans don't get enough exercise. If you don't stretch, your muscles tighten and don't work efficiently. If you don't move vigorously on a regular basis, the circulation slows, and the soft tissue doesn't get the nutrients it needs from the blood supply. You feel stiff and sore. Noxious waste by-products of broken-down cells are not carried away through the bloodstream, and they settle into scar tissue, which binds muscle groups together, making them work too hard.

Forced Speed

You are unique, and your ideal workpace is tied to your physical makeup. This variability can be likened to walking on a crowded sidewalk. Your stride depends on a combination of things, such as height, coordination, and energy. People with long limbs naturally outpace small people—unless that small person happens to be loaded with energy or the tall person has a languid gait.

People are routinely hired for typing speed (which is fallacious thinking, because "slow" typists may actually produce just as much work if faster typists take lots of breaks). A person whose pace is naturally slower has to strain to keep up with a fast person's pace. But not even fast typists should work at top speed every minute of the day. There's a natural rhythm to work: now fast, now slow, now take time to stop for a moment and chat with a coworker. If this rhythm isn't respected, the muscles fatigue; if they are not allowed to rest and recover, they become damaged.

Incentive Programs and Overtime

Incentive programs that link bonuses with speed and productivity are especially dangerous: Many people severely injure themselves by pushing beyond their bodily limits in order to make money. Overtime can be dangerous, too, because it further taxes muscles that are already tired and overused. Unfortunately, a lot of people are forced to work extra hours in order to make ends meet.

Excessive Monitoring

In her book *In the Age of the Smart Machine: The Future of Work and Power,* Shoshana Zuboff describes a phenomenon she calls the "information panopticon," which refers to the computer's ability to see and monitor every aspect of work, from counting keystrokes to ascertaining whether a task has been performed (and by whom).

Monitoring work activity is fairly widespread. According to the authors of *Healthy Work: Stress, Productivity, and the Reconstruction of Working Life,* Robert Karasek and Töres Theorell, the U.S. Office of Technology Assessment has estimated that in 1986 roughly 6 million workers were monitored by computer systems; such surveillance is often introduced "as a method of ensuring high output rate by making it impossible for employees to vary their pace or take occasional rest breaks." For some occupations, the percentage of such workers was 20% and growing. The authors note that "the invasion of personal boundaries leave[s] workers angry and resentful that their personal integrity has been undermined."

The trouble with having a computer rather than a human being keep watch over employees is that the computer doesn't have a heart. Before computers surveyed the workplace, employees could fudge if they needed more than the allotted time to complete a job. In his book *Technostress: The Human Cost of the Computer Revolution,* psychologist Craig Brod notes that, ideally, supervisors monitor their employees with understanding and empathy, but a computer does not take into consideration extenuating circumstances: "Where once a supervisor might know that an employee has just returned from a bout with the flu, and thus is having an off day, the computer cannot see beyond its standardized expectations of productivity."

Lack of Job Satisfaction

How people feel about their work can have a powerful effect on their health. If they feel good about it, they are less prone to stress-related disorders even if they have a relatively high stress load. If people don't feel good about their work, the opposite can be true: They can develop stress-related disorders such as headaches, ulcers, and insomnia or more serious problems.

Before the Industrial Revolution, people depended on cottage-based industries, farming, or hunting for sustenance. Because there was a direct relationship between a job well done and food on the table, people could take pride in how well they performed a job. A carpenter chose the wood with which to construct a table and applied hard-won skill to its creation. The table was his, from beginning to end. There was a sense of individuality in one's work, too. A studied eye could discern the author of unsigned work, for instance, from the way the stonemason had held the chisel while carving.

The inherent sense of purpose and fulfillment in work, the link between you and what you did, all but vanished with the advent of the "scientific management" developed by Frederick Taylor in 1911. In order to waste as little time as possible—and reduce the amount of motion, skill, and training necessary to do the work—jobs were divided into small parts and the pace increased. Taylorism removed decision making about how to do the work, "time-wasting" habits such as socializing with coworkers, and thinking about better ways to do the job—that is, all the things that make a job fun.

Taylorism also insists that everyone work at top speed all day long, an exhausting and depressing prospect. Instead of being able to decide for yourself how to approach a job and get it done, you were forced to do the same boring thing all day long someone else's way.

Company management liked Taylorism because it boosted productivity and helped ensure that no single employee became indispensable, thus allowing employers to control wages. The trouble is that when you deny people the ability to personalize their work, and when you take the challenge out of a job by oversimplifying it, you end up with bored, insulted employees who get no satisfaction from their jobs. Add to this the effect of repetitive motion on the body, and you get an unhappy, injured, and *angry* workforce. Angry employees are more likely to sue when they are hurt.

DEVELOPING RSI

RSI Comes on Slowly

If RSI happened with the drama of a broken wrist, people might be better off in the long run. They would take it seriously, go to the doctor, and allow themselves time to heal. It would be obvious to coworkers and bosses that they couldn't work until the injury healed completely.

But RSI creeps up on people. The body doesn't trumpet its distress—it whispers, and it doesn't even do that consistently. Very few people heed their symptoms until they've had several episodes of pain or incapacitation. And by that time, they've generally done serious damage to the soft tissues. They shrug off symptoms that should alert them to a problem.

This happens for three reasons:

1. Few people seem to understand that typing all day is physically strenuous—after all, they reason, you're just sitting at a desk.

2. The general public is ignorant about RSI, and people generally don't expect anything to go wrong with their hands, so their symptoms may be advanced before they seek medical help.

3. Many people have macho attitudes about pain and don't seek help until it becomes excruciating, or they have such poor body awareness they don't notice anything is wrong until it reaches an advanced stage.

However, people have usually noticed something odd long before they have episodes of pain or loss of motor control. One of my patients made an excellent point about differentiating between the transitory aches and pains of daily life and symptoms of RSI: "When I was a kid, the family doctor said you shouldn't be aware of your body," he recalled. "He meant that when the machine functions normally it doesn't squeak. I'm not talking about body awareness in the sense of feeling alive, but that if you wake up and you are aware of your arms, it's your body signaling a dysfunction somewhere." The onset of RSI can begin with merely having an increased awareness of your hands without being able to pinpoint exactly why.

If the symptoms are left untreated, eventually all kinds of crazy things happen to people: Their fingers no longer do what they are told; they get shooting pains down their arms; their fingers start going numb; or they have bouts of unaccustomed clumsiness or involuntary muscle spasms. At this point they start seeing doctors.

Recovery Takes Time

When they receive a diagnosis of repetitive strain injury, people usually feel relieved to know what is wrong. They figure if they stop the offending behavior, which for many people is linked to computer use, their hands will go back to normal in a few days. But the damage from overuse occurs after months and years of abuse, and the body is slow to forgive. Recovery takes time, and people need to learn to change certain behavior—for life. Others, who wait too long or are improperly diagnosed or treated, may become permanently disabled.

THE PROBLEMS WITH CURRENT TREATMENT

All Doctors Are Not Equally Informed about RSI

A large number of my patients have expressed great exasperation in connection with seeking treatment for RSI. They tell me their doctors treated them like children; the exam was too short; the doctors were arrogant or cynical, or told them to do something inappropriate, such as go back to work when they were in too much pain to touch a keyboard. My patients describe coming in for their appointments—frequently in great pain and panic-stricken—only to be seen for ten minutes and sent home because the doctor "couldn't find any cause" for the injury. Or they are diagnosed with something they don't have: I have seen too many young people who had needless surgery for carpal tunnel syndrome because, as their doctors put it, "there was nothing else to do." If there is nothing left to do, unnecessary surgery is certainly not the answer.

Even if the diagnosis is correct, incorrect attribution of the cause can frustrate recovery. One woman was livid because her doctor said her problem arose from lifting up her child instead of the long hours she spent at the computer for her job. "I'm sick of people telling me it's from picking up my child. I *wasn't* picking her up—I was at work. The only women I know who have problems picking up their kids are women who work with computers."

In a similar situation, when one of my patients told his doctor that his right hand hurt, the doctor said to use the other one. This simple-minded approach backfired, however. "I switched hands, and then my left hand started to hurt," he complained. Refraining from computer use will not even necessarily relieve the pain of a severely injured person—that may require months of physical therapy. Furthermore, if you don't use good technique, you'll reinjure yourself when you return to work.

Many Doctors Are Skeptical about the Existence of RSI

I never believed in RSI until I got it.

— RSI patient

It is almost impossible to keep abreast of all advances in medicine, so a physician's ignorance about RSI is understandable. Callous dismissiveness is not. Complex as it is, the anatomy of RSI is easier to explain than the current controversy surrounding it. Why do some members of the medical profession doubt that RSI is computer related or even view the existence of

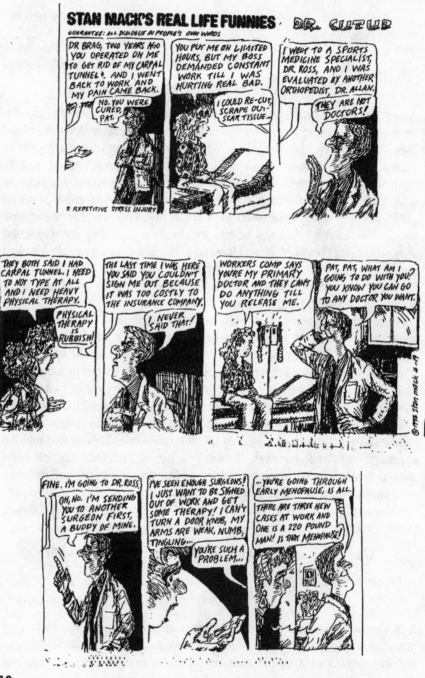

RSI with skepticism? Despite the staggering number of computer users who are afflicted with various maladies of the hand and forearm, these skeptical doctors hold that symptoms cannot be attributed to computer work, an assertion akin to the medical experts who said lung cancer could not be attributed to cigarette smoking. They say aching and discomfort are a common reaction to diligent work, which is a questionable assertion; work should not cause pain. They also maintain that the problem is due to other activities. But if you examine the patient and find that he is utterly sedentary aside from spending hours on end at the computer overworking his hands and arms in a cramped and awkward position, and has injured the muscles used to operate the keyboard, doesn't it seem logical to suspect that work might be the cause? Common sense dictates that this is the first place to look.

Instead, these physicians claim RSI exists only in the minds of the patients. An Australian study of an RSI epidemic by Yolande Lucire suggested that it was a form of conversion hysteria. Lucire holds that repressive forces of society are internalized and block the expression of unacceptable sexuality, anger, desires to be cared for, and other needs that are in conflict with the demands of the environment. So, she reasons, these powerless and dependent people, "who cannot otherwise express their righteous rage at their supervisors, employers and spouses, resort to the use of their exquisitely symbolic pain and incapacity as a mode of communication of their distress."

According to another Australian study, the abundance of women involved was characteristic of epidemic hysteria, especially in an occupational setting. Aside from the fact that RSI afflicts a large number of men, epidemic hysteria couldn't account for self-employed people with RSI who work in isolation. Furthermore, a lot of my salaried patients are well-paid, highly motivated, and gifted people who hold powerful positions. They bear absolutely no grudge against their employers, who in turn value their services.

This phenomenon is not hysteria; it has a perfectly rational explanation. The epidemic occurs in three waves. In the first wave, the more severely injured people can't work. Seeing their coworkers go out on disability scares a second wave of people who are having chronic, but not disabling, symptoms. The third-wave people come in with minor symptoms because they've identified what happened with the first two waves and want to catch it early. So RSI is not really mass hysteria. This epidemic in a communal workplace has a rational explanation. And every good doctor knows ways to identify employees who are malingering, so there's no reason to mislabel this as hysteria.

Other health-care providers accuse patients of taking advantage of Workers' Compensation and disability payments. A few people probably do try to defraud Workers' Compensation, but since the money amount is lower than what can be made working, that argument doesn't hold in most cases. No rational person would prefer disability payments to being able to use his or her hands.

An Open Mind Is Essential to the Practice of Medicine

Many doctors protest that the very term *repetitive strain injury* is misleading, because there is no scientific basis proving that repetitive work causes tissue strain or injury. Perhaps there could be a more descriptive term, but in the meantime, why wait for epidemiological studies on causation before you treat someone for an injury?

If cynicism about RSI were contained only in the minds of physicians, it would be lamentable, but it wouldn't hurt anyone. Such doctors, however, send injured patients home because they "can't find anything wrong," or think "it's all in your head." If that person continues to work, ignorant of the damage done by using poor technique, he worsens the injury, and it will keep getting worse until—and unless—he finds a doctor capable of making an accurate diagnosis and taking him off the injury/reinjury treadmill through treatment and retraining.

Doctors are certainly entitled to their opinions and healthy skepticism, but it would help if they would keep an open mind to the possibility that repetitive work could cause repetitive strain injuries. Failing that, they might at least treat the injuries they see. There are many objective signs of RSI, such as those described in Chapter 7. When RSI is correctly diagnosed, it is apparent that patients aren't making up their symptoms. When it is not correctly diagnosed, patients run the risk of permanent injury.

PREVENTION IS THE BEST MEDICINE

Once people have damaged their soft tissues, they are always at greater risk for reinjury or chronic bouts of RSI. RSI can be prevented through education, ergonomics, and enlightened job design. RSI is far easier to prevent than cure, and if people don't heed this warning, all of society will eventually pay because its tax dollars will have to support permanently disabled people who otherwise would have led productive and self-sufficient lives.

CHAPTER 2

A Commonsense Approach to RSI: The Seven-Point Program

Common sense is the knack of seeing things as they are, and doing things as they ought to be done.

— Calvin E. Stowe, 1802–1886

Your RSI resulted from a combination of factors, which could include your posture, your work habits, the type of work you do, your workstation arrangement, and your hereditary makeup. This book will show you how to prevent and recover (if you are not too severely injured) from RSI using a commonsense approach. You will learn how to correct or cope with each contributing factor, one by one.

The same basic principles apply to both preventing and recovering from RSI, so if you don't have RSI but are worried about getting it, you can still use this program. Though treated separately here, the guidelines are all equally important and are meant to be integrated simultaneously. No book can replace the guidance of a physician or physical therapist, so bear in mind that you should learn to master these principles under professional guidance.

THE SEVEN POINTS

Physician

An accurate diagnosis forms the cornerstone for recovery. You should see a physician to find out if you have a serious underlying medical problem such as diabetes, thyroid disease, arthritis, or another condition (such as Lyme disease or pregnancy) that could cause or complicate RSI. These issues are covered in more detail in Chapters 4 and 6.

13

Pain Management

The first step toward recovery is getting out of pain. Pain management begins with physical therapy. Muscles and other soft tissues need to move to remain healthy. Deep tissue massage remodels scar tissue and allows muscle more range of motion. Stretching and strengthening exercises help keep muscle supple, toned, and pain free.

Eventually you will learn how to relieve pain yourself. Icing sore or painful areas, for instance, is an excellent way to reduce pain and inflammation, and it is generally more effective than taking drugs (see Chapter 11).

Posture

Good posture is essential to preventing RSI, but few people understand what the term means. Posture is a dynamic, not static, concept: It means keeping bones aligned through movement and stillness, with muscles at their optimum length instead of too tight or overstretched. This balanced use of muscles affords ease of movement and freedom from pain, *not* the tension that comes from holding yourself stiff like the stick figures in a handout on ergonomics (which many people actually try to do!). See Chapters 4 and 10 for more on posture.

Preventive Exercises

Thousands of repetitive movements cause microtrauma to muscle tissues, which leads to inflammation. The debris left by inflammation creates scar tissue, which binds down the muscle and in turn stresses tendons. Stretching can reverse the injury process and promote healing.

Muscles work in unison, so through physical therapy you must learn to stretch and strengthen corresponding muscle groups so they can work harmoniously. Tight muscles on one side of a bone cause the muscles on the other side to overstretch and weaken. Your physical therapist must stretch the tight areas to allow the proper range of motion. However, this now-relaxed muscle will stay in its new framework only if the corresponding muscles are tightened by strengthening exercises. You must do these exercises faithfully to keep everything in balance and remain in shape for your work. See Chapter 11 for suggested exercises.

Positioning

Proper positioning refers to both the correct configuration of the chair and desk and the correct angling of the body to the computer monitor and keyboard. You must set up your workstation to fit your own physical dimensions. See Chapter 15.

You must also learn to position your hands correctly at the keyboard. This retraining of typing technique is crucial to rehabilitation and prevention of reinjury. You can have a state-of-the-art ergonomic situation, but if you don't know how to type safely, you're still at risk for RSI (see Chapter 16).

Pacing

You can help prevent injuries—and ward off flare-ups if you're already injured—if you learn to pace yourself. If you are not injured, take a 5- to 10-minute break from typing for every half hour that you work. One break per hour should include stretching; the other could be spent doing nonkeyboard activities. If you have RSI, see the instructions on pacing in Chapter 16, page 183.

Patience

After suffering the relentless abuse of thousands upon thousands of key-strokes, the body is slow to forgive and heal, yet many people expect an overnight cure. Once they realize the extent of their injury, they want to be well immediately, which is understandable, and it's quite a disappointment when they find out how long healing takes.

The slowness of recovery can be highly frustrating, so when people feel a little better, they try to catch up, push themselves to work too hard, and wind up having a relapse. The danger here is that reinjury can be worse than the original injury and can happen much more quickly. Relapses are very discouraging to people, too.

Recovery may take months or years, so patience forms the backbone of the program. See Chapter 10 for more on patience.

THREE OTHER POINTS

Remember That RSI Is Invisible

RSI is a hidden disability. If you were wearing a cast on your arm, someone might offer you a seat on the bus, or give you a hand with your packages, or open a door for you. But RSI doesn't show, and sometimes people will be skeptical about your inability to use your hands, or the pain you feel. Even doctors don't believe you sometimes. See the coping advice on pages 140–142.

Listen to Your Body

No one—not your doctor, not your physical therapist, and not your employer—knows how you feel as well as you do. If you have an instinct that something may be harmful to your hands, listen to that instinct. Try to analyze what activities bother you, and trace your pain to its source and avoid aggravating your injury. An RSI log is particularly helpful here (see page 114).

Use Your Head

No one can give you all the answers about RSI, and there is no substitute for your own common sense. If something about your treatment troubles you, don't assume you're wrong and everyone else is right. Ask questions, keep an open mind, and look for the answers that make the most sense to you.

TWO USEFUL TERMS

I've tried to use very little medical jargon in order to make my points as clear as possible. However, there are two medical terms that couldn't be replaced with lay terms, because substitutes were inaccurate, vague, or misleading. Just exactly what do people mean by a bent wrist, anyway? Are your fingers facing up or down? Doctors use precise medical terms to avoid confusion. Only two of them are used here, so either memorize them or flag this page for quick referral.

Dorsiflexion means putting your hand in the position policemen use to stop traffic, with the palm at an upright angle to the wrist. An easy way to remember dorsiflexion is to think of pushing open a *door* with a dorsiflexed hand (see Figure 1.) Figure 35 on page 178 illustrates the proper way to position your hand at the keyboard.

FIGURE 1   Improper Keyboard with Dorsiflexion.
Resting the hand on the edge of the desk or wristpad causes dorsiflexion (hands bent upward at the wrist), a major source of injuries. Raising the far end of the keyboard worsens this problem by increasing the angle of hand and wrist.

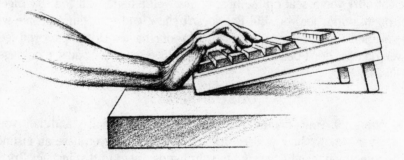

FIGURE 2 Radial Deviation.   **FIGURE 3 Neutral Wrist Position.**   **FIGURE 4 Ulnar Deviation.**

When you type, you should keep your hand in a *neutral* position.

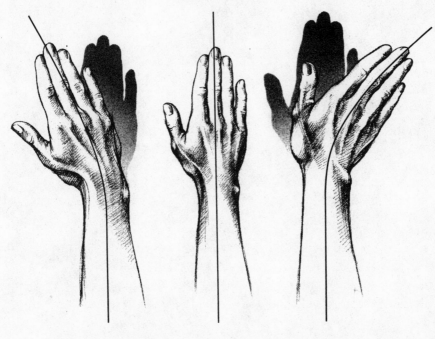

Ulnar Deviation refers to the position in Figure 4, with the hand bent from the wrist in the direction of the ulna, the bone on the same side of the arm as the pinkie finger. Think of a pair of windshield wipers that move in opposite directions: When they go toward the outside of the car, they are in ulnar deviation. When they go toward each other, they are in *radial deviation* (see Figure 2), because the *radius* is the bone on the same side of the arm as the thumb. Figure 33 illustrates what ulnar deviation looks like at the keyboard.

When you type, your hands should be in neutral position as in Figure 3. See also Figure 34 (page 177) which illustrates what this looks like at the keyboard.

CHAPTER 3

Symptoms of RSI

Repetitive strain injury acts like a cunning mugger: It sneaks up on you without your being aware of it. When first seeking treatment, many patients realize that they had experienced warning signs long before and wish they had acted sooner.

To complicate matters, the pain associated with RSI moves around. One day you might feel discomfort in the shoulder and the neck, the next day it is in the upper back, and the day after that it travels down your arm.

This migratory quality of RSI is probably caused by unconscious postural compromises people make to protect a painful area. If their shoulder hurts, they might work their arms a little harder. The shoulder feels better the next day, but then the arm hurts. People often do not deduce that their symptoms are connected to their posture. Rather than perceive these feelings as the subtle beginning of RSI, people typically attribute it to sleeping wrong or aging or, as one patient put it, "Gee, all this time I thought pain was just part of the job!" Some forms of RSI can be painless, so be careful to read the checklist before deciding you don't have a problem because you aren't in pain.

Symptoms of RSI differ from person to person, depending on the site of the injury. Even if you type for as little as two or three hours a day, if you experience any of the signs below, you should consult a qualified physician. Not every ache or pain indicates that you have RSI, but if you have several symptoms and the gut instinct that all is not well, you owe it to yourself to check it out. You probably wouldn't have bought this book if you weren't worried. If you experience headaches or eyestrain, see Chapter 9. Discuss other problems that you feel are computer-related with your physician or rehabilitation therapist.

RSI affects the entire upper extremity, that is, the neck, shoulder, upper back, upper arm, forearm, wrist, and hand. As Michele Semler, a physical therapist at the Miller Institute who works with many RSI patients, put it, "I rarely just work on one area, such as the forearm. It's usually the forearm, the hands, the shoulder, and the neck." Pain or other symptoms in your neck, shoulders, upper back, or forearms all can signify RSI, so don't assume that if you don't have wrist or hand pain you don't have a problem.

Furthermore, pain or numbness in your hands or wrists could stem from problems in your neck or shoulder.

Warning Signs of RSI

Pain

Sustained, or chronic, pain of any kind is a sign that something is wrong, and for people with RSI, it can occur almost anywhere in the upper extremity. Don't dismiss pain as unimportant. The pain of RSI manifests itself in a multitude of ways. It can be burning, aching, or shooting. It can be restricted to small sites, such as fingertips, or settle in over a diffuse area such as the forearm. You may feel pain when you work, or feel it when you don't even move. The pain can wake you up at night.

But remember, you can have severe RSI *without* experiencing pain; tremors, clumsiness, and numbness can all be symptoms of RSI.

Fatigue or Lack of Endurance

If you find yourself getting worn out easily or notice that you just can't type as long as you once could, take it seriously. "I can do something, but I can't do anything for very long," said one patient. For reasons that are not well understood, lack of endurance haunts RSI patients long after they have reached a pain-free state. One temporary secretary suffered for days after simply holding an umbrella during a parade one afternoon.

Weakness in the Hands or Forearms

RSI can cause general weakness in the hands and forearms, which makes it extremely difficult to do things most of us never think twice about, such as lifting wet laundry out of the washing machine, pulling the lid off the teakettle, or lugging a shopping bag.

Tingling, Numbness, or Loss of Sensation

Tingling, a feeling that your hand or arm "fell asleep," and diminished sensitivity of touch can be signs of nerve damage.

Heaviness

A feeling of heaviness, sluggishness, or fatigue is a symptom of RSI. Some patients say their hands and arms feel like "dead weight."

Clumsiness

It's normal to drop things or lose your grip once in a while, but if you keep shattering glassware, or find yourself having to concentrate actively on something that should be automatic, such as holding on to your coffee mug (or needing both hands to do so), you might have RSI.

Difficulty Opening and Closing Hands; Stiffness

If you have difficulty opening and closing your hands or wake up in the morning with your hands cramped into claws, it could indicate a problem.

Difficulty Using Hands

Difficulty with normal activities such as opening doors, chopping vegetables, snapping your fingers, picking up small objects, and turning faucets on and off is a common sign of RSI.

Lack of Control or Coordination

The feeling that your fingers aren't doing what you wanted them to, or that you have lost control of them, could be a by-product of RSI. In one extreme case, a man found himself very embarrassed when, upon shaking hands during an introduction, his own hand traveled up the wrist of another man; he had lost that much motor coordination.

Cold Hands

Chronically cold hands, particularly the fingertips, can signal a distorted nerve function.

Heightened Awareness

Just being vaguely aware or hyper-aware of a body part can be a clue that something is wrong. "My hand never feels normal," one patient said. "My fingers feel sluggish. They don't feel like my own," reported another. This super-awareness is not accidental. Your body may be trying to warn you that something is amiss by drawing your attention there. How do your hands feel when you wake up in the morning? If they are painful or sore, it could mean you have RSI.

Hypersensitivity

Tenderness to the touch, the feeling that you're wearing a bracelet when you aren't wearing one, or other supersensitive sensations can indicate RSI. Some people get a burning sensation when the skin over a tender muscle is lightly stroked. Women report having more RSI-related pain before and during their menstrual periods.

Heightened sensitivity after minimal use of your hands or arms can also indicate RSI. You should tell your doctor if something as minor as opening a jar has triggered an episode of pain.

Frequent Self-Massage

Self-massage is an instinctive attempt at healing. Someone who constantly rubs an area over her neck, shoulder, wrist, hand, or forearm or finds herself shaking out her hands because they have gone numb could very well have RSI.

Tightness

Sympathy Pains

RSI sufferers can have their own symptoms triggered if others with RSI start talking about their pain. There is an extreme sensitivity to pain; the thought of the keyboard, or having to push open a heavy door, can also trigger pain.

Do You Have RSI?

If you find yourself modifying your daily behavior in any of the ways listed below, you should make an appointment with a competent physician for an evaluation. Curtailing your daily activities can be a warning sign of RSI. Early diagnosis can be your key to recovery; ignoring symptoms could lead to permanent loss of the use of your hands.

Do you:

_____ Avoid using the injured hand?

_____ Do things with your nondominant hand that used to be easier with your dominant hand (dialing the telephone or punching your codes into the automatic teller machine at the bank with your left hand when you are right-handed, or vice versa)?

_____ Use your forearm, feet, or shoulder, instead of the injured hand, to push open doors, or find yourself shaking out your hands because they have gone numb?

_____ Avoid wearing or buying certain kinds of clothing because it is too difficult to put them on?

_____ Change shopping habits because you can't carry as much as you once could?

_____ Keep dropping things?

_____ Find you can't peel or chop food?

_____ Stop playing sports you once enjoyed or change sports?

_____ Experience trouble tying ties or buttoning collar buttons?

_____ Have trouble hooking bras or putting on jewelry?

_____ Stop wearing heavy bracelets because your wrists are tender?

_____ Have trouble with keys or brushing teeth?

_____ Feel overly protective of your hands (refuse to shake hands, or worry someone will bump into them on the street)?

_____ Not trust the injured hand (hang on to the handrail, subway strap, or bus pole with the "good" hand)?

_____ Have trouble holding a book or newspaper?

Many people tend to disregard or deny clear messages that they have a problem. They say they don't type enough to have RSI, yet their posture and technique is so abominable that the typing they do can give them symptoms.

Jane Bear-Lehman, who teaches occupational therapy at Columbia University and has a private practice in New York City, remarked on some of the subtle and not-so-subtle cues her RSI patients ignore. "They tell me they were unloading the dishwasher and dropped all the glasses. One woman told me she used plastic cups at home, yet she didn't find that odd. They can't hook their earrings any more. Tying neckties is a problem for men; women don't wear (or buy) certain blouses because they can't fasten the buttons. They'll change sports, or stop doing the sports they enjoyed. But they don't think they have RSI!"

Don't ignore symptoms. They are your body's way of signaling distress. If you have to curtail your daily activities because your hands, shoulder, neck, or forearms hurt, you've got a problem. See your doctor. The sooner you get help, the better chance you have of preventing RSI from becoming permanently disabling.

CHAPTER 4

Assessing Your Risk for RSI

Risk factors for RSI fall into two categories: intrinsic factors, which are those caused by body structure, disease, and work habits; and extrinsic, or external, factors, those caused by the workstation configuration, type of work, work environment, or keyboard. You can't get an accurate picture of RSI by looking at the ergonomics of the workstation without also taking the person's medical history into account. Both must be considered.

A better practice is to look at the *whole* person and take a thorough history, so I ask a lot of questions: Are there diseases or traumas that could have precipitated or worsened RSI? Are you taking any medications? How is your general health?

Here, even a standard medical history does not suffice: How do you carry yourself when you stand and sit? How aware are you of pain? What kind of mental outlook do you have on life? People are driven by distinct hopes, fears, and needs, and two people with similar physical types might respond to the same work demands differently because of their personality; this must be taken into account. Some clues for pent-up tension can be as subtle as the way people breathe: Shallow breathers hold tension in their necks, which aggravates RSI. People who clench their jaws have the same problem.

Once you have been evaluated for physical or psychological predisposition toward RSI, your doctor should consider your environment: Are you being pushed by a slave-driving boss? Is your work environment relaxed or competitive? Must you meet constant deadlines, or are you free to work at your own pace? Must you work two jobs or overtime to make ends meet?

Finally, people with no physical predisposition for RSI can injure themselves because of the way they use their hands at the keyboard. All of these factors need to be considered.

YOUR TYPING STYLE

Typing style far outweighs other factors in causing RSI. I have videotaped hundreds of computer users at work, and hardly any of them had safe technique. Instead, they unwittingly used certain injurious styles and postures which I have grouped into the following categories.

Resters

Resting the hand on the edge of the desk or wristpad is nearly universal among computer users. This causes dorsiflexion (hands bent upward at the wrist), a major source of injuries.

Here is an image to help you understand what happens when the hand is held in dorsiflexion. (See Figure 1 on page 16.) If you think of the tendon as a rope attached to a heavy bucket, and the bone and ligament as the edge of a roof, it's easy to understand how easily the tendon could become frayed from repeatedly dragging the bucket up over the edge of the roof. This shearing action is the equivalent of continual dorsiflexion. On the other hand, if you were standing on level ground and pulled the bucket straight toward you over a well-balanced pulley system, there would be little friction. This unstressed movement is the equivalent of a neutral wrist position (see Figure 3 on page 17, Figure 34 on page 177, and Figure 35 on page 178).

NOTE: Many ergonomists mistakenly encourage people to rest their hands on a wristpad while they work, because it keeps the wrist in a more

FIGURE 5 Proper Sitting Position for Typing.
Here the spine is correctly aligned, with the ears in line with the shoulders and hips, the shoulders hold the chest open, the arm supports the hands above the keyboard, and nothing is strained.

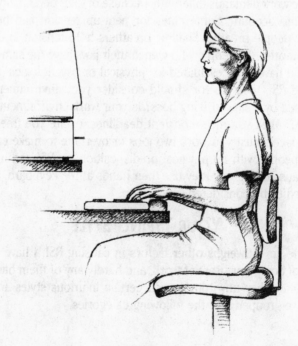

neutral position. *Don't do this.* This posture forces the small tendons of the fingers to do work the big shoulder joints and muscles should do. It also encourages ulnar deviation, because resters tend to reach for keys keeping the heel of their hand planted on the wristpad instead of properly moving the whole hand over the keyboard in a neutral position. Let your hands float over the wristpad as you type (as in Figure 35 page 178), and rest them on its cushioned surface *only when you are not typing.* See Chapter 16 for proper typing technique.

Leaners

Leaners type with their elbows on their desk or the arms of their chairs. This habit can lead to nerve damage, among other things.

Loungers

Loungers sit with their spine slumped in the back of their chair, and often compound this disastrous posture by putting their feet on the desk. Slouching compresses the spine, causing low back pain. It also throws the head forward, which can lead to neck and shoulder problems. (See Figures 5 and 6 for proper and improper positioning.)

FIGURE 6 Improper Sitting Position for Typing.
Here the spine is slumped, the shoulders contract forward, and the wrists are in dorsiflexion. This posture strains the neck, shoulders, back. forearms, and wrist.

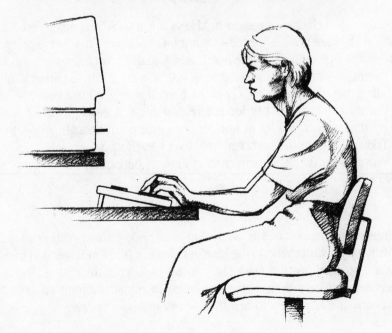

Clackers or Pounders

People who hit the keys far harder than necessary are "clackers." They make such a racket you can hear them halfway across the room. If you multiply 1½ ounces of pressure by the number of keystrokes you do per day, as much as 1½ tons of pressure could go through your fingers. Therefore, the gentler the touch, the better.

One of my patients came in complaining of pain and tingling in his finger-tips and joints. It was easy to see why: He really slammed his fingers into the keyboard. His nerves were probably battered from all that pounding, causing the tingling sensations he complained about.

He knew he should use a light touch when he typed, but he had a tough time changing his habit. Under pressure, he would hit the keys as hard as ever. "May I offer my insight into this?" he volunteered. "A long time ago, I made a psychological link between hitting the keys very hard and doing very good work." The challenge for him, then, was to change the attitude that caused the damaging style.

Another man admitted he pounded the keyboard when he was angry, and because he was working at a job he considered beneath him, he felt angry most of the time. However, taking it out on the keyboard only hurt him. He needed to channel his anger into another, safer direction.

Pressers

A subgroup of clackers, pressers hold keys down until their fingers go white, and—if they are double-jointed—their joints collapse. This undue pressure strains the tiny tendons of the hands and forearm muscles.

During a videotaping session, one editor whose job required a lot of scrolling held a cursor key down so hard her finger blanched. She was obviously angry at the key for not responding fast enough; she was also angry that there was a lot of work at her job and not enough people to do it. Taking it out on the keyboard only hurt her, though.

People who do sustained scrolling have to be careful not to press too hard.

Pointers

Pointers—self-taught typists who hunt and peck instead of touch-type—usually rely instinctively on the strongest fingers (the forefinger and middle finger), so they are the least likely to be hurt from their style. Pointers, because they have their forearms poised in midair to hunt all over the keyboard, are less likely to rest their wrists or ulnar deviate.

FIGURE 7 Improper Keyboard Technique.
"Pointing" with the middle finger, which can cause the other fingers to contort, and thumb and pinkie extension can lead to forearm tendinitis and deQuervain's disease.

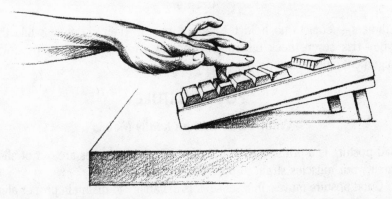

Pointing can be dangerous if you hold your other fingers in a contorted position as in Figure 7. So if you hunt and peck, keep your fingers curved.

Thumb or Pinkie Extenders

People who keep thumb or pinkie or both lifted as they work are at great risk for forearm tendinitis and deQuervain's disease. If you want to understand the risk involved with this position, hold your hand out as though to type, stick your pinkie in the air, and try wiggling the remaining fingers. It will be much more difficult, because the tendons must fight each other to keep the pinkie aloft while the other digits move. Do the same thing with your thumb, noticing the sensation of strain in the web of your hand and forearm. Now try wiggling your fingers with all of them curved and relaxed. It will be effortless.

NOTE: Working with the thumb relaxed is particularly difficult. See Chapter 16 for exercises to help you learn how.

Grippers

Using a mouse instead of a keyboard can be dangerous, because rather than the fingers sharing the workload, the entire burden falls on a single digit of one hand. To make matters worse, the table may be too high, so muscles in the shoulder and neck are needlessly tensed. Trackballs present danger because they require so much wrist and finger motion, and they should be used with great care.

Grippers are people who grip the mouse too tightly or use too much force when they click. The mouse should be held loosely, keeping the wrist in neutral position; when you click, don't raise your finger higher than necessary.

See page 182 for instructions on how to handle your mouse.

Cradlers

Cradlers—people who hold the phone up with their shoulder while they type—risk severe neck disorders. Cradling also throws the spine out of alignment, and makes proper positioning difficult.

YOUR POSTURE

What Good Posture Really Means

Bad posture is a primary risk factor for RSI; if your bones are out of alignment, your muscles strain to hold you erect.

Good posture moves, in a sense. It is the ability to maintain proper alignment of the bones and length of the muscle through motions. This does *not* mean holding yourself stiff like the stick figures in an ergonomics handout, as many people think. That kind of rigidity actually hurts your body. Most people's idea of good posture stemmed from an order to "Stand up straight!" issued by their mother or gym coach. This is unfortunate, because good posture really means balanced use of muscles, ease of movement, and freedom from pain, not the tension that comes from holding yourself stiff. In order to accomplish this, though, muscles need to be stretched and toned and must work in a balanced way.

Slouching, Shifting, and Fidgeting

Like any animal, humans naturally move, shifting their weight from foot to foot, or relaxing and straightening the spine. This natural stress reaction has been toned down by civilization; it is considered rude to stretch or yawn. But fidgeting is good for you, because it keeps muscles from becoming overloaded. During a retraining session, one woman leaned back in her chair, then caught herself. "Is this okay?" she asked. The answer was yes. She had been leaning back, absorbing a discussion about keyboard technique. She wasn't typing, and she would be sitting properly in a moment or two, so it was good for her to rest the muscles that had been tired.

Postural Syndrome

Most people wouldn't consider poor posture a serious medical problem, but it can become just that over time. Poor habits can lead to what is called *postural syndrome*—a nagging, diffuse pain or discomfort.

Postural Dysfunction

Postural syndrome degenerates into a postural dysfunction when the musculature becomes frozen in bad positioning because the muscles have become unbalanced. Profound physiological changes have occurred, so you can't realign your own joints well enough to correct alignment without outside help. Once postural dysfunction has reached this stage, it is hard to reverse. You can see this with people whose habitual posture is out of whack: They hold one shoulder higher than the other, or their back is swayed, or they can't hold themselves erect for very long without intense effort.

Psychological Factors of Posture

Postural habits begin with early childhood, so by the time people become injured, they've already developed deeply ingrained patterns of holding themselves. Psychological factors can affect posture, too: A shy person may habitually tense his shoulders or jut out his jaw, so unlearning this habit may mean presenting a new face to the world, something the person may resist. Some women might be extremely self-conscious about sitting up straight if they feel it puts their breasts on display. One very tall man confessed that he slouched in his chair because he hated his job so much he was trying to make himself smaller, as though he weren't there. Another big man habitually ducked his head so as not to intimidate smaller people.

Postural Compensations

People have varying degrees of body awareness, and it can take some people a long time to comprehend what the physical therapist tells them. They may slouch, sway their backs, or carry one shoulder higher than the other without being conscious of it. Destructive posture feels "normal" or "good" to them, even though it is actually malalignment.

Postural problems can have a number of causes. One of my patients was honest enough to show us how she really sits at the computer: with one foot tucked under her buttocks or resting on an open file cabinet drawer. She acknowledged that her posture wasn't great, but she explained that "it makes my back hurt less" to sit that way. She had broken her back in a car accident, displacing a vertebra. She needed to have physical therapy to get her muscles back in balance so she could sit comfortably in less stressful positions. If you don't address these problems after your body suffers a trauma like that, you are likely to compromise your posture to get "comfortable" the way this woman did. See Chapter 10 (page 92) for more on posture.

YOUR JOB

The kind of work you do can be a risk factor for RSI. Jobs that primarily require typing, such as data entry, telephone information, or 911 dispatch work, are very dangerous because they do not allow enough rest time. The mental stress associated with these jobs is great because people have little or no control over their work. Continuous, machine-paced input creates a hazard for the hands.

YOUR ENVIRONMENT

Crowding

Your work environment can contribute to RSI by raising your stress level. Smoky, noisy, or cramped quarters; inadequate ventilation; harsh lighting; and dust can be powerful if subtle stressors. One man complained bitterly about not ever being capable of getting comfortable in his chair because it was too close to that of his coworker, who bumped into him all day long. When you work 8 to 12 hours a day in this sort of situation, the stress really adds up.

Physical crowding can also cause psychological cramping because your personal space is being invaded. Employees whose boss stands over their shoulders while they type carry an enormous burden of strain.

Moving from Workstation to Workstation

Many people complain about being forced to move from workstation to workstation at their job; it is often impossible to get a good ergonomic fit in this situation. There is also a psychological factor, as pointed out by Charley Richardson, director of the Technology and Work Program at the University of Massachusetts, Lowell: "People make their workstation their home. Then the boss says, 'We're going to move you around' and you don't have a home any more." In addition to the physical inconvenience, an emotional instability occurs.

YOUR GENETIC HERITAGE

Anatomy is destiny.

— Sigmund Freud

In a way, RSI begins with your genetic heritage. Your DNA dictates a number of things: a tendency toward leanness or plumpness, your bone structure, and the likelihood you may contract certain ailments that might predispose you to RSI, such as arthritis, diabetes, or thyroid disease.

Double-jointedness

A very common, but mostly overlooked, predisposing factor for RSI is hypermobility of the finger joints, or double-jointedness. Instead of holding firm when a key is struck, the finger joint collapses. This causes the wrists to bounce up and down. It may sound minor, but if the wrist bends thousands of times a day, the tendons in the fingers, wrist, and forearm are strained.

Some people try to compensate for this tendency to collapse by contracting the two muscle groups that bend and straighten the fingers at the same time. This "co-contraction" exhausts the muscles.

Obesity

It may not be obvious why being overweight can underlie repetitive strain injury, but obesity can be a major contributing factor. Obese people frequently must force their hands into ulnar deviation just to get around their own physical mass to put their hands to the keyboard. Extra pounds also add to the weight the muscles must support just to hold the forearms to the keyboard. Overweight people are more likely to have other conditions that affect their general health, too.

Slenderness

People with slender or slight builds are especially at risk for RSI because they don't have enough muscle mass to support the heavy work they are doing. You wouldn't use a spoon to dig a ditch; you'd use a shovel. So smaller muscles fatigue and get injured more easily than bigger ones do.

This does *not* mean that you should gain weight or become a bodybuilder (though strengthening exercises do help). It simply means you will have to be more careful than someone with big muscles.

Age

Age alone does not cause RSI, but older operators can develop RSI simply because they've been at the job longer. The average age of my patients is 39. However, as keyboard work proliferates, this number could go down.

Sex

Women tend to get RSI at a higher rate than men do, but RSI is hardly a woman's disease. Women are simply more susceptible because they generally have smaller muscles than men; computer work requires a lot of strength, so big muscles give men the advantage. In addition, hormonal changes from pregnancy, menopause, and gynecological surgery can cause swelling, which in turn can put them at risk for carpal tunnel syndrome.

This higher proportion can also be partially attributed to the large numbers of women who work in jobs that require repetitive movements of the hands and arms: secretaries, data entry processors, telephone operators, and cashiers.

Long Fingernails

Long fingernails prevent you from curving your fingers to strike the key. Flat-fingered typing causes co-contraction (tensing two muscle groups at once), and holding any muscle rigid for too long exhausts and damages it.

Other Diseases

Alcoholism, rheumatoid arthritis, high blood pressure, diabetes, thyroid or kidney disease, gout, or pregnancy can predispose people to RSI for various reasons.

Drugs

Certain drugs, such as oral contraceptives, blood pressure medications, and nonsteroidal anti-inflammatories, cause water retention. If the soft tissue swells, it can aggravate nerve compression problems, such as carpal tunnel syndrome.

YOUR PERSONALITY, ATTITUDES, AND DRIVES

To truly understand repetitive strain injury, you need to know a lot about human nature. Our attitudes can shape our health as surely as our environment and genes.

Machismo and RSI

Macho attitudes about pain and weakness permeate our culture, and this refusal to acknowledge pain can lead to disaster. Pain is there to tell you something is wrong, and you should listen to it, not ignore it.

Women can have this attitude, too, but it is still more common among men. Though men are less likely to get RSI than women, they are often severely injured, probably because they wait so long to get treatment while they try to tough it out.

When a man develops RSI, it can devastate him. Some men feel emasculated by their disability and become so severely depressed that they consider suicide.

Macho attitudes can also lead to sexist claims, such as labeling it a "woman's disease." RSI can happen to anybody.

Driven Behavior

One of my patients could partially attribute his RSI to internal drive: "I tried to get the work out as fast as possible. I always bought the fastest equipment possible," Brad recalled. He took pleasure in the speed afforded by the light touch of the keyboard.

Brad typically worked 8-, 10-, or 12-hour days and some Saturdays. He noticed odd symptoms, but "I just didn't pay attention. I felt I slept wrong." This went on until he was unable to work, he had difficulty feeding himself, and—perhaps the ultimate loss—he was unable to drive.

Brad was the kind of employee managers love—highly motivated, good at what he did, and proud of it. But he needed to learn to balance his physical needs with his inner drive.

Shyness

People who don't assert themselves are at higher risk for RSI because they may not have the nerve to state their needs about work pace or ask for a new chair or other ergonomic equipment. As one patient put it, "When I tell my boss I need a special table, I think, how about the other thousand employees who work here? I'm one of the lowest employees." The patient asked me for a note, which is a good way to handle this problem.

Some people are too shy even to ask their physician for help. Dr. Joseph DePietro, the medical director for the *New York Times*, said he treated a woman who had quietly borne great pain before she sought help. By the time he saw her, her condition had progressed to the point where it was nearly irreparable, and she will probably never return to her former position. "Suffering in silence is not uncommon," said Dr. DePietro.

These same people court reinjury because their pacing and technique go out the window when they have pressure on the job. If you are too shy to tell your employer what you need to do to get better, get a doctor's note spelling it out. Your doctor should state specifically what you are allowed to do so that your employer understands the nature of your injury.

THE CORPORATE CULTURE

Fast Pace, High Pressure

If you work in a fast-paced environment, or if someone in a superior position pushes you, it can be very difficult to take breaks, much less work at your own pace.

One woman who worked as a financial analyst reported overhearing a member of senior management say, "You have to give these people more unrealistic deadlines. It doesn't look good—people aren't working nights or weekends."

The analyst said this about her job pressures: "If you get reasonable deadlines, they give you too many other things to do at the same time, which amounts to the same thing," she said. "If you have no physical problems, you can stay day and night and do it. But I can't work furiously any more—I need to take breaks and exercise."

In her environment, people don't even chat with each other, much less stop to stretch. "If I exercise, everybody sees," she said. It is a shame that she senses coworkers' disapproval because *she's stopped working for a moment to take care of her health.*

The Economy

A bad economy breeds RSI, because instead of hiring enough staff, employers are firing people and pushing those who remain to work too hard. Many people fear layoffs, which adds to job stress. "My big fear is permanent disability. I don't know how to do anything else," said a high-level newspaper editor.

Another patient, like many other people, became injured trying to make ends meet as a word processor. "They weren't paying me enough so I worked 62 hours a week for six months," she said. "Four other word processors are also affected. No one has said anything because they're afraid they'll lose their jobs."

THE ROLE OF STRESS

Hans Selye, whose book *The Stress of Life* made *stress* a household word, defined it as the rate of wear and tear on the body.

Many people misunderstand stress to be a terrible bane that must be removed from their lives, but stress is far more complicated than that. First of all, the term *stress* encompasses happy excitement as well as terror, so *distress* is a better word for what most people understand as stress. Secondly, no one can avoid stress in life, and stress really isn't so terrible *if you have a positive way to cope with it.*

Stressors can be internal (such as worry) or external (such as disease or trauma). When you put a high-strung worker in a situation loaded with anxiety, say a reporter on deadline with a breaking news story or a legal secretary who must finish typing the brief by noon, the reaction happens like this: The body doesn't know the difference between a true life-or-death situation (such as having a mugger pull a knife on you) or something essentially harmless (like having your boss lose her temper with you). Your body responds to this threat by releasing adrenalin and corticoids and you feel agitated. The cycle of stress is the same for happy or sad things: You get excited, and then you have a "depression," a let-down phase that Selye tells us keeps us from going at top speed for too long. There is a tug-of-war between tension and relaxation that must be balanced.

You can have stress in your life without adverse effects if you have positive coping mechanisms. These can be as diverse as vigorous exercise, napping, meditation, or going fishing. People who cope with pressure by abusing drugs, alcohol, or nicotine compound the problems of stress; people who have positive coping strategies will be able to handle hard times with ease.

In the book *Healthy Work*, which addresses stress-related heart disease, authors Robert Karasek and Töres Theorell point out that low-status workers who bear heavy psychological demands but lack the freedom to make decisions about their work are at far greater risk than executives with a high degree of control over pacing. They compare the jogger, who faces high levels of stress but is self-paced and in control, with the assembly line worker facing a speedup. People forced to do overtime work in uncontrollable and boring jobs—more often the case with women—will suffer more strain than those who do overtime work in stimulating, controllable jobs.

An unhealthy combination of stressors produces a dangerous chain reaction in the adrenal system. Stress can kill, as in the case of heart disease, but there are other unpleasant "diseases of stress": high blood pressure, ulcer, and even cancer. Someone joked that the most effective form of stress management can be summed up in two words: Say no.

The best stress reducer, then, may be quitting your job; unfortunately, this is hardly a viable option for most people. Karasek and Theorell note that "most of the solutions currently advanced to reduce stress—relaxation therapies, for example—address only its symptoms. Little is done to change the source of the problem: work organization itself." The authors hold that the solution to job-related stress lies in the transformation of the workplace.

This is a noteworthy goal. But perhaps you should also take stock of your situation, and consider whether you should really be doing the work you're doing, or make career changes that allow you more control over your life.

YOUR LIFESTYLE

You live badly, my friends. Is it really necessary for you to live so badly?

— Anton Pavlovich Chekhov

Fatigue

If you don't sleep well, or take enough breaks during the day, your body doesn't have the chance to recuperate from exertion. Tired muscles are more prone to injury.

Diet

After a decade of interest in good health, American health habits have reverted to a dismal pre-1980s state, according to a recent poll. "Americans continue to get fatter," lamented Humphrey Taylor, president of Louis Harris & Associates. "We are the fattest nation on Earth." A survey of health habits showed that Americans were eating more fat and salt, fewer vegetables, and less fiber-containing foods. Sixty-six percent of those questioned were overweight. "For doctors in the country, this report is terribly disturbing," said Dr. Todd Davis, executive vice-president of the American Medical Association. "It means Americans are not willing to accept responsibility for their own well-being." Some of these health habits could increase longevity.

A balanced diet is essential to good health. Your body must obtain enough of the right kind of nutrients to function well. If you abuse it with a high-fat, high-salt, high-protein diet, you court heart disease, high blood pressure, and obesity. High-salt diets can also cause water retention, which can aggravate nerve compression problems.

Conversely, you can do yourself a favor by eating well. Consider the value of antioxidants, which are thought to clean up waste created by overexertion in muscle tissue. Including foods containing antioxidants in your diet could help you heal more quickly. (See page 80 for more on antioxidant vitamins.)

Caffeine

Most people associate caffeine with coffee drinking, but tea, cocoa, and soft drinks (and several over-the-counter medications including pain relievers, cold preparations, and weight-control aids) contain it.

Caffeine is viewed as an ergogenic aid; that is, it increases the ability to do work. This happens because caffeine stimulates the brain and diminishes fatigue during prolonged exercise. Caffeine stimulates the central nervous system, increases the heart and respiratory rates, and increases urine output. It can also upset the rhythm of the heartbeat and cause headache, irritability, depression, and sleeplessness.

If you don't sleep well you are at greater risk for injury because of fatigue. Don't take over-the-counter stimulants to stay awake for work. Instead, get some more sleep.

Eliminating caffeine from your diet may cause withdrawal symptoms such as headaches; if you stop drinking coffee, do so gradually.

Alcohol

Alcohol has a potent effect on the body. It disturbs REM (rapid eye movement, or dream) sleep, which means that you may not be as refreshed from sleep as you should be to work safely. If you drink too much, you may wake up agitated and tired. Alcohol aggravates soft tissue injury, because it causes dehydration. By reducing sex hormones, it can lead to depression and pain.

Alcohol use can complicate reflex sympathetic dysfunction (page 58) because in large doses it destroys endorphins and other natural painkillers and eventually makes the body dependent on outside chemicals for substances it used to create on its own. Alcohol can also set up a vicious cycle, as Hooshang Hooshmand points out in *Chronic Pain: Reflex Sympathetic Dystrophy Prevention and Management:* "Alcohol is an unstable and volatile source of energy that is rapidly utilized by the nerve cells . . . alcohol becomes addictive like sugar . . . for an already defective malnourished and damaged brain."

Recreational Drugs

Drug abuse worsens chronic pain because your body stops manufacturing its own painkillers. You wouldn't use these drugs if you were an Olympian athlete because they would adversely affect your performance. The same things applies to your performance at the keyboard.

Smoking

In addition to other well-known risks, smoking exacerbates RSI because nicotine hampers good blood circulation. If your blood doesn't flow well, waste products can settle into scar tissue instead of being carried away in the bloodstream. In addition, smoking replaces oxygen with carbon monoxide. Smoking is a risk factor for cervical spondylosis, a neck problem.

Good circulation brings food and oxygen to the muscles. If your muscles don't receive food and oxygen, they tire easily. Don't smoke to cope with stress; find something better, such as exercise, breathing techniques, or meditation.

Sedentary Behavior

Nearly three out of five adults in this country lead sedentary lives, according to a report in the *New York Times*. This inactivity is associated with a host of problems, including back pain, heart disease, and obesity, which is a risk factor for RSI.

EXACERBATING ACTIVITIES

When you tally your risk factors, don't forget the other things you do with your hands during the day. Some people tally only the number of hours they use a computer at work every day, forgetting to mention the hours they spend at a home computer, working or playing video games. Driving, another common activity, requires a lot of sustained exertion and can be a very stressful activity. One of my patients gripped the steering wheel of her car so tightly that she developed trigger finger (see page 51).

If you hold the pen in a death grip while you write; do a lot of carpentry, gardening, sewing, or other needlework; lift weights or participate in other sports with heavy hand use; or play a musical instrument, ask your physician or occupational therapist how to modify those activities so it doesn't worsen your RSI.

RISK FACTOR CHECKLIST

You are at risk for RSI if you have a combination of the following risk factors:

_____ Use a computer more than 2 to 4 hours a day
_____ Have a job that requires constant computer use, especially heavy input
_____ Don't take frequent breaks
_____ Are loose-jointed
_____ Have poor posture
_____ Have poor technique
_____ Don't exercise vigorously and regularly
_____ Work in a high-pressure environment
_____ Have arthritis, diabetes, thyroid disease, or another serious medical condition
_____ Keep your fingernails long
_____ Smoke or drink excessively
_____ Weigh more than you should

Any of the above can be problems, but the more you have, the higher your risk.

PART II

DIAGNOSIS AND TREATMENT OF RSI

CHAPTER 5

Getting an Accurate Diagnosis

Listen to the patient. He's giving you the diagnosis.

— attributed to Sir William Henry Osler (1849–1920)

Because computer-related RSI is a relatively new development, some doctors are not prepared to diagnose it, much less treat it. My patients frequently complain that it took several visits to various physicians before their condition was properly identified. Many cases are misdiagnosed as carpal tunnel syndrome when the real problem is tendinitis or deQuervain's disease. Even if people get an accurate diagnosis, many of them are not informed about technique retraining, pacing, or workstation improvements, which are required if people expect to continue to work safely. Too often, patients have told me a doctor dismissed their quandary with a shrug and said, "Don't type so much." This advice does not help someone who makes a living using a computer.

To properly diagnose RSI, your physician needs a good understanding of how the hand works, the diseases and conditions discussed in Chapter 6, and knowledge of what constitutes good ergonomics. Your doctor also must know *your exact working conditions*. He should look at what you

41

are required to do at your job, analyze both the extrinsic and intrinsic ergonomics—that is, both your workstation and your posture and physical makeup—and help you make adjustments to work safely. If your doctor doesn't have an adjustable chair, keyboard, and table in the office so you can replicate your workstation, you should bring photos or a videotape of yourself working. If time permits, arrange for your physician to visit your workplace.

You might be able to receive the assistance of an ergonomist through your state's occupational safety department, or your company's safety department, if it has one.

After pinpointing the problem, your physician should prescribe a multi-faceted treatment program. This includes:

- Physical therapy to stretch and strengthen the affected muscle groups
- Learning to control pain, take adequate short rest breaks and recognize the body's warning signals to stop working
- Retraining your typing technique so you don't get caught in a cycle of reinjury

If you are improperly diagnosed, or if you are not retrained to type properly, RSI will worsen while you continue to work, and you risk permanent injury.

When to See a Doctor

The earlier you see a doctor, the better your chances of recovery. Don't wait until your symptoms are severe, because the longer you wait, the more likely it is that your condition will worsen. (See Warning Signs of RSI, page 20.)

What Kind of Doctor to See

RSI can be a baffling disease, affecting neck, shoulder, forearm, and hand, as well as bone, nerve, and muscle. Ailments in these areas can be treated by orthopedists, hand surgeons, neurologists, occupational medicine doctors, physiatrists, rheumatologists, internists, and family practitioners. The first problem facing many people is deciding what kind of doctor to see.

Most of my patients saw at least six different specialists before they were properly diagnosed, and they often describe an exasperating odyssey. Typically, people try both traditional medicine and alternative treatments. First, they see their chiropractor or acupuncturist. When that doesn't solve the problem, they try their general practitioner. Then they see a rheumatologist, or orthopedist, then a hand surgeon, then an occupational health physician. Because there is an uneven awareness in the medical community about RSI, any one of these doctors could be the right one for you—but any one of them could also be the *wrong* one. For instance, people go to orthopedists because they have musculoskeletal problems, but if that orthopedist is not knowledgeable about soft tissue injury, the problem may be underestimated, ignored, or misunderstood.

HOW TO CHOOSE A PHYSICIAN

For many people, seeing a doctor involves taking a leap of faith. People generally feel powerless in the face of illness because they don't know what's happening in their bodies and must rely on a doctor to tell them. The traditional view of the doctor as a kind, wise, and heroic practitioner of healing arts has been replaced by an image of greed and indifference, and many people think the most they can hope for in a physician is competence. But physicians of the old school exist, and you can find one to treat you.

If you already have a family doctor you like, that's a good place to start. Physicians with specialties sometimes tend to see all problems in terms of their own practice; a surgeon might be more likely to recommend surgery, for instance. A family practitioner may be able to help you herself or refer you to the appropriate specialist.

Other sources for referrals are knowledgeable friends, RSI support group members, or recommendations from a facility that is known for interest in occupational medicine or one that treats musicians or athletes, who often have problems similar to computer users. Keep asking. If the same name keeps coming up, chances are that person might be very good.

Big-Name Doctors May Not Be Worth the Wait

Think twice about going to a famous doctor. Sometimes you'll wait six months for an appointment with such a physician, then be kept waiting four hours in the reception area, only to have the doctor spend five or ten minutes with you. You can't get good care in five minutes.

The doctor's reputation may be richly deserved, but if the doctor is indifferent or inaccessible, then someone equally skilled and less well-known, but more concerned, would be a better choice.

The Clinical Examination Is Important

Technological advances cut both ways: For all our modern wizardry, nothing can replace a good hands-on clinical evaluation. Nowadays, though, many doctors put machines between themselves and their patients. Any testing should support a clinical diagnosis, not vice versa. This means the doctor should talk to you, listen to you, and touch you (test your muscles, for instance) before tests are ordered. Of course, many doctors automatically recommend expensive, and sometimes painful, tests such as the electromyogram (EMG) that may be unnecessary because they fear that one day they will be asked in court why they *didn't* perform such-and-such a test.

Evaluate the Physician

Here are some ways to help you evaluate your physician.

Does your doctor listen well?

The most important part of any examination is taking a thorough case history. Your doctor should really listen to you and ask questions based on your answers. Doctors should be good detectives, eliciting important facts that will lead to an accurate diagnosis. Watch out for doctors who let a nurse or assistant take your history—they may not hear for themselves the subtle cues that could lead to important diagnostic findings.

If your doctor intimidates you or doesn't give you a chance to say what's bothering you, find one with more patience. You deserve to be treated with sensitivity.

Is your doctor sympathetic to RSI?

Many doctors won't see a connection between computer work and your injury. Vincent Rossillo, a Manhattan attorney who represents a large number of RSI claimants, put it this way: "A lot of people say their doctor tells them they have tennis elbow, but they don't play tennis. These people do the same type of repetitive motions, eight hours a day, for years."

Furthermore, some doctors are downright hostile to the notion of RSI because they think it is based on subjective symptoms—that is, it's all in the head. There has been little research on soft tissue injury (which is involved in most RSI cases), perhaps because it does not lead to profitable surgical operations such as a carpal tunnel release. In addition, treating these injuries is labor-intensive for the physician; a thorough examination takes an hour and a half. Obviously, if you use computers and think you were injured doing that, it is best to find a physician who understands how your job activities could relate to your symptoms and will help you work safely rather than one who dismisses work as a possible cause.

Will your doctor be your advocate?

Once your doctor accepts you as a patient, she must be prepared to become your defender, because RSI patients are constantly besieged by their insurers, employers, and Workers' Compensation for notes, opinions, and documentation. Your doctor must be willing to oversee every aspect of your recovery, from ensuring that work modifications are acceptable and your workstation is properly adjusted to getting your employer to allow you to work at a reasonable pace, take rest breaks, and sit in a decent chair. (See page 160 for more suggestions.) If your doctor won't be your advocate, find another one who will. You will probably have a long relationship with your doctor, so make it a solid one.

Is your doctor competent to treat RSI?

You may think the world of your physician as a person, but if he doesn't understand the subtleties of RSI, you'll need another doctor. For guidelines on how to evaluate this, read Chapter 6 carefully before you go for your appointment.

Does your doctor accept Workers' Compensation cases?

If your RSI is work-related, find out if the doctor accepts Workers' Compensation cases *before* you go.

Many doctors refuse Workers' Compensation cases for a number of reasons. Workers' Compensation requires them to do a lot of paperwork and occasionally testify at hearings. If the case is contested, they may not get paid. On top of that, they usually don't receive their standard fees.

Although this can make finding a doctor more difficult, the reluctance is understandable: If your doctor or physical therapist treats you, and Workers' Compensation refuses to pay for that treatment, the doctor or therapist may have to absorb the loss, which is difficult considering the cost of running a practice.

Do you trust your doctor?

It doesn't matter that your physician has sterling credentials and an impeccable reputation, or that everyone you know sees her. If you don't like or trust that doctor for any reason, find someone else. This also applies to other health practitioners, including physical and occupational therapists and masseurs. You must be able to trust the person treating you in order to make good progress.

QUESTIONS PATIENTS ASK

Will I get better?

Yes—if you've come in for treatment before permanent damage has occurred. But it will take time. It will require a lot of patience and persistence on your part, too, because you will have to do your exercise routines faithfully, undergo extensive physical therapy, and learn to pace yourself carefully.

Some people injure themselves so severely they will never regain full use of their hands. The best outcome may be reduction in pain with limited use of the hands.

Will I come back 100%?

If you haven't been severely injured, you'll eventually be almost as good as new. But soft tissue injury can take many months, even years, to heal, and once the tissue is damaged, it always remains fragile. You can never go back to old habits without risking pain and reinjury. Remember, endurance will be the last thing to come back.

How long will it take?

There are no pat answers, but you should think in terms of months or even years. People are usually out of acute pain and will have regained some strength and flexibility after three to six months of therapy, but many still have flare-ups even years later. Much of your recovery will depend on you and your circumstances. If you can afford to stop working, and then work at your own pace when you return to your job, you'll probably fare better than someone who can't or doesn't want to take time off. In addition, people who respect their bodies' pain signals will do better than those who don't.

If you've been seriously injured with RSI, you need to be careful with your hands for the rest of your life, as you would with similar injuries.

Is there anything I shouldn't do?

Don't work through pain. Don't try to strengthen your hand or forearm muscles by lifting weights. Don't do chin-ups or push-ups. Talk to your occupational therapist about modifying exercise equipment—attaching cross-country ski machine straps to your upper arm instead of your hands, for instance. For other advice, see Chapters 11, 12, and 14.

WHAT TO TELL YOUR DOCTOR

Tell your doctor about past surgeries or injuries; any diseases or disorders you have; and any medications, prescribed or otherwise, that you take. If you're upset emotionally because of your injury, say so. Perhaps you can get Workers' Compensation to cover psychotherapy.

Fully describe your job, your workstation, and the conditions under which you perform. Bring videotapes or photos of yourself at your workstation.

Measure the height of the seat of your chair and desk so your doctor can judge the relative safety of your setup.

DURING YOUR OFFICE VISIT

Ask questions about anything you don't understand concerning your diagnosis. Be sure to get guidelines on what to do and what to avoid doing.

Make sure your doctor knows exactly what you do at your job. If you continue to work, get any instructions about what you should or shouldn't do in writing (see page 160).

BE A SMART MEDICAL CONSUMER

Finding a good doctor need not be a matter of luck. Choose your health-care professionals with the same care and discretion you would exercise with any other product or service. You are entitled to a thorough examination. You should be allowed, and even encouraged, to ask questions, and you are entitled to receive answers in plain English. Remember, it's your body—and your money.

Checklist

_____ Does your doctor listen well?
_____ Is your doctor sympathetic to RSI?
_____ Does your doctor accept Workers' Compensation cases?
_____ Will your doctor be your advocate?
_____ Is your doctor competent to treat RSI?
_____ Do you trust your doctor?

Ideally, your doctor should meet all of these criteria. If you checked all of the above, you probably have found a physician with whom you can adequately tackle RSI.

If not, maybe you can accept the lack of certain qualities in your physician because you are happy in other areas. Otherwise, you should keep looking.

CHAPTER 6

Classifications of Repetitive Strain Injury

Repetitive strain injury is an umbrella term for several cumulative trauma disorders caused by overuse of the hand and arm. The tendons, tendon sheaths, muscles, ligaments, joints, and nerves of the hand, arm, neck, and shoulder can all be damaged by repetitive movements. These soft tissue injuries fall into three basic categories: tendon, ligament, and muscle disorders; nerve disorders; and neurovascular disorders, which affect both nerves and blood flow.

RSI manifests itself according to individual physical weaknesses or areas vulnerable to faulty work habits or workstations. Some people have pain in their shoulders, necks, or wrists. Other people don't have much pain, but experience extreme weakness or clumsiness.

This chapter presents the major diagnoses of RSI. These descriptions are meant to give you general information about symptoms and the possible cause of your symptoms. When you read them, they may sound similar to each other. Don't try to diagnose yourself. You need a skilled doctor to decide what form you have.

One caution: Some doctors know little about RSI. This is not to suggest that you second-guess your doctor, but if you mention your symptoms to your doctor and he says there is nothing wrong with you, or that it is normal to feel pain when you work, and is unwilling to pursue the cause of your symptoms, seek another medical opinion. RSI is serious, and if you are not properly diagnosed, you risk permanent injury.

CARPAL TUNNEL SYNDROME IS NOT THE ONLY KIND OF RSI

One of the most irritating misconceptions about RSI is that RSI is synonymous with carpal tunnel syndrome. This belief most likely arose in the beginning of the epidemic, when the press relied on doctors who didn't understand all the manifestations of RSI. Carpal tunnel syndrome is relatively rare among RSI patients; deQuervain's disease, which affects the thumb and thumb-side of the wrist, is a far more common problem in my experience. According to the National Institute for Occupational Safety and Health's study of RSI at US West Communications, 15% of all employees had tendon-related disorders, but only 1% had carpal tunnel syndrome.

Annoying as it is, this inaccuracy wouldn't be so awful if it didn't have such serious consequences. However, because people don't know about the other, more common kinds of RSI—and they don't have the symptoms of carpal tunnel syndrome they read about in the news—they put off seeking treatment. They don't realize anything serious is wrong.

Here are some common kinds of repetitive strain injury, with descriptions of symptoms.

NOTE: You should also be aware that it is not uncommon for people to have five or six different problems at once. For example, a person may have forearm tendinitis and myositis, deQuervain's disease, a nerve impingement in the neck, and a lack of mobility in the shoulder. Such a person lumps symptoms together and presents an array of diagnostic possibilities that need to be sorted out and treated separately.

MUSCLE AND TENDON DISORDERS

Tendinitis

Tendons connect muscles to the bone. Tendons consist of tissue that has little stretch or rebound, so if you tax your tendons beyond their strength by overuse or hold your hands rigidly for hours on end, tiny tears occur in them, leading to tendinitis. Friction from overuse can cause inflammation and contribute to tendinitis. Because of the tendons' anatomic function, they are highly susceptible to repetitive strain injuries.

In general, larger muscles do the big work and smaller tendons perform fine actions. The extensor muscles of the forearm, for instance, are only about the size of a pencil in circumference. When people rest their wrists on the edge of the desk while they work, they overload the tiny muscles and tendons of the hand and forearm. Computer work requires the assistance of powerful muscles of the shoulders and back, but these muscles cannot be engaged if people rest their wrists while they type.

Muscle Damage

Muscle damage can be caused by overwork. Myofascial damage is characterized by tenderness in the muscle that is worsened by stretching and pressing. One of the most common findings in RSI, myofascial tenderness often goes unrecognized by physicians, particularly when it occurs in the flexor and extensor (top and bottom) muscles of the forearm.

If you have myofascial pain, your muscles will feel sore to the touch, at rest or during use. People often complain of burning sensations while they type. If left untreated, this tissue can swell, press on nerves, and lead to scarring and worse pain.

Tenosynovitis

In areas where tendons must curve around bones or change directions, they often pass through tendon sheaths. These protective coverings perform the same function as the housing of a speedometer cable or a pulley. The inner wall of the tendon sheath secretes a slippery substance, called synovial fluid, to lubricate movement. If the tendon and the sheath rub together, the resultant irritation is called tenosynovitis. If this friction continues, the sheath can eventually respond with an overproduction of fluid. If the tendon sheath swells and won't fit comfortably into areas where the anatomy is already snug, such as the carpal tunnel, nerve compression can result.

Stenosing Tenosynovitis

Stenosing tenosynovitis occurs in chronic cases. Here the tendon moves with great difficulty through the sheath, causing very painful conditions such as deQuervain's disease or trigger finger.

DeQuervain's Disease. DeQuervain's disease occurs where the tendon and tendon sheath merge at the junction of the wrist and thumb (see Figure 8). Patients with this syndrome feel acute pain when they move their thumb or perform an action that requires a twisting motion, such as wringing out a dishcloth. People who hold their thumbs up while they type or hit the space bar with too much force are prone to deQuervain's disease. Because it occurs in the wrist, it can be misdiagnosed as carpal tunnel syndrome.

Trigger Finger (Flexor Tenosynovitis). Trigger finger is the locking of a digit in a bent position. It occurs when a nodule or ganglion cyst forms on the tendon. This bump gets caught in the sheath, and the finger locks, so the person must straighten it with the other hand. The pain associated with trigger finger can be bad enough to make someone cry.

Trigger finger can occur on any finger but is most common in the ring finger and thumb.

FIGURE 8   DeQuervain's Disease.

DeQuervain's disease is tenosynovitis at the base of the thumb
that affects the abductor pollicis longus and the extensor pollicis
brevis. It is characterized by the inflammation, thickening, and
tenderness of these tendons and their sheaths. (Reprinted with
permission from *Scientific American Medicine*, Section 15, Subsection XII. ©1992 Scientific American, Inc. All rights reserved.)

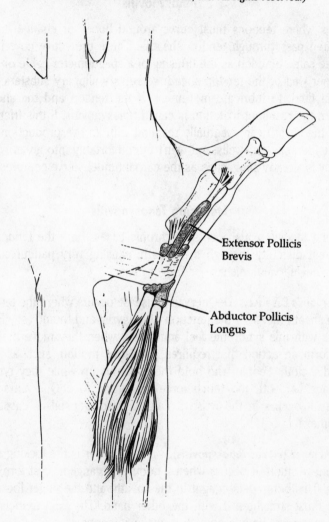

Extensor Pollicis
Brevis

Abductor Pollicis
Longus

Shoulder Tendinitis

Bicipital Tendinitis. Bicipital tendinitis occurs where the biceps muscle inserts into the shoulder joint. You'll feel uncomfortable when you raise your arms to the front if you have bicipital tendinitis, which can occur as a result of poor posture (shoulders slumped forward), or repeatedly moving the arm over a surface too high or too far away, such as moving a mouse on a high table.

Rotator Cuff Tendinitis. The rotator cuff is a group of muscles and tendons near the shoulder joint that turn the arm in and out and move it away from the body. Discomfort reaching into a hip pocket or hooking a bra can indicate rotator cuff tendinitis. Rotator cuff tendinitis is associated with overusing the arm with the elbows "winged" away from the body, as they are when the keyboard is too high.

Forearm Tendinitis

Flexor Carpi Radialis Tendinitis. Flexor carpi radialis tendinitis is another affliction affecting the wrist. It produces tenderness at the base of the thumb muscle. The flexor carpi radialis muscle pulls the wrist down, so this form of tendinitis may come from hitting the space bar too hard.

Extensor Tendinitis. Extensor tendinitis affects the muscles used to straighten the fingers. Pain appears on the top of the hand near the wrist, probably because the hands are held for prolonged periods in dorsiflexion.

Flexor Tendinitis. Flexor tendinitis affects the muscles used to bend the fingers. Pain usually appears in the fingers. You can develop flexor tendinitis from excessive finger motion or gripping a mouse.

CERVICAL RADICULOPATHY

Because this condition occurs most often in people who hold the phone with an upraised shoulder while they type, I call cervical radiculopathy the "phone shoulder syndrome." This seemingly innocent behavior can be observed everywhere, from kitchens where homemakers stir stews or chop vegetables, to cramped phone booths where salespeople write in appointment books. You've probably done it yourself a hundred times at the keyboard.

Don't do it. Cervical radiculopathy is a compression that commonly affects the C5 and C6 or C6 and C7 cervical discs in the neck and makes head movement extremely painful. If you have this injury, you also might feel weakness in the shoulder and upper arm, and possibly have numbness in your fingers. See page 172 for an example of how dangerous this injury can be.

Poor posture, such as habitually keeping the neck craned forward, can contribute to cervical radiculopathy.

Epicondylitis

There are two major forms of epicondylitis: lateral (outside the elbow) and medial (inside the elbow). Commonly known as tennis elbow, bowler's elbow, or pitcher's elbow if the pain is on the outside of the elbow—or golfer's elbow if the pain is on the inside—this condition usually results when the desk is too high for the person using it, forcing her to raise her elbow. Dorsi-flexion or ulnar deviation can also contribute to tennis elbow. Patients with epicondylitis can experience extreme pain while attempting to straighten their arms or contract them against resistance. The area over the elbow is tender to the touch.

There appears to be a high incidence of epicondylitis among mouse users.

Ganglion Cysts

Ganglion cysts occur on the tendon, tendon sheath, or synovial lining of the joint. An ovoid bump forms beneath the surface of the skin. Ganglion cysts are often associated with aching or weakness and usually appear in four places: on top of the hand, just above the wrist; on the nailbed; on the crease of the far finger knuckle; or on the palm side of the wrist. Although ganglion cysts are not usually dangerous—unless they compress a nerve—they are a sign of wear and tear, and they can indicate the presence of RSI.

According to Vern Putz-Anderson, author of *Cumulative Trauma Disorders: A Manual for Musculoskeletal Diseases of the Upper Limbs,* ganglion cysts used to be called "bible bumps" because people used bibles—then the most available book—to smash them. Now this can be accomplished surgically. There is no harm in leaving them alone unless they are compressing a nerve.

TUNNEL SYNDROMES

Nerves that pass through "tunnels" created by bones, ligaments, and other tissue can be damaged if the surrounding tissue swells and presses on them. Tunnel syndromes can occur at many sites throughout the body, and there are several that affect the movement of the arm. Symptoms of tunnel syndromes include pain, muscle weakness, and numbness. With tendinitis, pain generally worsens with movement and gets better with rest. But with tunnel syndromes, pain can be constant, becoming worse with movement. Because swelling occurs more at night, the pain also tends to wake people from sleep.

Three nerves can be involved with RSI: the median (middle), radial, and ulnar.

MEDIAN NERVE DISORDERS
Carpal Tunnel Syndrome (CTS)

The carpal tunnel is a bracelet formed by bone and tough ligament just below the wrist at the heel of the hand (see Figure 9). Through this rigid structure pass nine finger tendons, connective tissue, arteries and veins, and the median nerve, which conducts impulses from the brain down the arm to the thumb, forefinger, middle finger, and half the ring finger. Excessive up-and-down wrist and finger movement (like that used for striking computer keys) eventually irritates the synovium (the lining

FIGURE 9 Carpal Tunnel Syndrome.
Carpal Tunnel Syndrome involves the entrapment of the median nerve in the canal that encloses the nerve and several flexor tendons and is formed by bones of the wrist and the transverse carpal ligament. Traumatic thickening of the flexor tendon sheaths can compress the median nerve. (Reprinted with permission from *Scientific American Medicine*, Section 15, Subsection XII. ©1992 Scientific American, Inc. All rights reserved.)

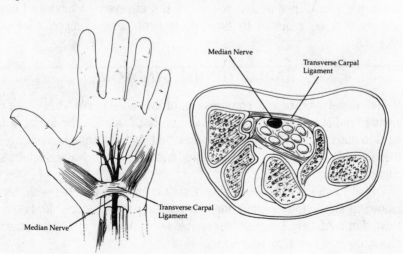

Median Nerve

Transverse Carpal Ligament

Transverse Carpal Ligament

Median Nerve

of the carpal tunnel), causing swelling. Because the carpal tunnel can't expand to accommodate this swelling, the pressure on the median nerve causes the numbness and tingling associated with carpal tunnel syndrome.

Carpal tunnel syndrome usually creeps up on people. In addition to numbness or tingling in their fingers, patients complain of soreness and pain that wakes them up at night, a cardinal sign of carpal tunnel syndrome. They note a loss of power in their grip or find themselves constantly dropping objects.

Other Causes of Carpal Tunnel Syndrome

Carpal tunnel syndrome is associated with many other medical conditions often involving fluid retention, such as pregnancy, use of oral contraceptives, diabetes, and thyroid disease, so it is important for your doctor to take a comprehensive medical history when making a diagnosis, then treat the primary cause of CTS. Lyme disease is also associated with carpal tunnel syndrome.

Dynamic and Passive Carpal Tunnel Syndrome

I separate carpal tunnel syndrome into two categories: dynamic (related to repetitive motion) and passive (caused by rheumatoid arthritis, diabetes, hypothyroidism, or other diseases).

Surgery

Symptoms of CTS can come and go, and it often responds very well to aggressive physical therapy and retraining. But in severe or advanced cases, surgery may be required to avoid permanent nerve damage. (See page 78.)

Radial Tunnel Syndrome

Radial tunnel syndrome is compression of the radial nerve. One of the first signs of radial tunnel syndrome is pain on both sides of the forearm. It is hard to make a fist. The fingers are weakened, with the thumb usually being the last digit affected. Twisting motions, such as wringing a washcloth, can aggravate symptoms.

Radial tunnel syndrome can be mistaken for, and co-exist with, tennis elbow; in fact, another name for it is resistant tennis elbow. It should be treated immediately, because irreversible nerve damage can occur. In some cases, doctors recommend surgery.

PAIN ON TOP
NOT ON BOTTOM

PAIN IN
THE ELBOW

ULNAR NERVE DISORDERS

Sulcus Ulnaris Syndrome

When you understand what the individual words mean, sulcus ulnaris syndrome doesn't sound quite so threatening. *Sulcus* means furrow, or groove, and *ulnaris* refers to the ulna, a bone of the forearm. Thus, sulcus ulnaris syndrome is a problem in a bone groove near the inside of the elbow.

People with a shallow groove on the ulnar bone (the funny bone) who lean on their elbows at work are likely to develop sulcus ulnaris syndrome. This posture presses on the ulnar nerve and cuts off the blood flow. Symptoms include loss of sensation, numbness, tingling, muscle atrophy, and a clawlike appearance of the ring and pinkie fingers.

In severe or advanced cases, surgery to move the nerve may be required to avoid permanent nerve damage. (See Chapter 8.)

Cubital Tunnel Syndrome

Also known as *flexor carpi ulnaris muscle syndrome,* cubital tunnel syndrome strikes people who work with their elbows bent at right angles for long periods of time, as in the case of computer workers. It involves a possible nerve entrapment that occurs in the underarm over the pathway of the ulnar nerve. Symptoms include loss of sensation, numbness, tingling, and muscle atrophy. Cubital tunnel syndrome can be confused with epicondylitis.

Guyon's Canal Syndrome

Guyon's canal syndrome, also called ulnar tunnel syndrome, is compression of the ulnar nerve in the wrist in another tunnel, near the carpal tunnel. Ulnar tunnel syndrome may be associated with trauma to the ulnar nerve caused by repeated radial deviation or dorsiflexion. Symptoms include numbness in the ring and little fingers and difficulty grasping. Pain may be aggravated by both dorsiflexion and flexion (bending the wrist up and down). When someone has both cubital tunnel syndrome and Guyon's canal syndrome, it is called a "double crush."

PROBLEMS INVOLVING NERVES AND CIRCULATION

Thoracic Outlet Syndrome

In order to remain healthy, muscles must receive a plentiful supply of oxygen-rich blood. When both arteries and nerves are compressed, the

/ALSO WING of THE BACK
& ACHILLES

result is thoracic outlet syndrome, which includes a number of ailments. Signs of this problem include pain in the entire arm and numbness, coldness, and weakness in the fingers, hand, and forearm. Symptoms can be provoked by carrying heavy loads, or working with the arms elevated, such as when styling hair or writing on a blackboard.

Raynaud's Disease or Phenomenon

NO

One of the primary symptoms of Raynaud's disease or Raynaud's phenomenon is cold, pale fingers due to blood vessel constriction. There can also be painful sensitivity, tingling, and numbness. Secondary Raynaud's phenomenon occurs in the presence of an underlying disorder, such as trauma, rheumatoid arthritis, thoracic outlet syndrome, and connective tissue disorders such as systemic lupus erythematosus. In primary Raynaud's phenomenon (sometimes called Raynaud's disease), predisposing causes are absent.

Primary Raynaud's phenomenon is five times more common in women and usually affects both hands. Secondary Raynaud's phenomenon does not have such a high female percentage and affects one hand more often than both.

If you have Raynaud's disease, don't smoke, because this constricts the blood vessels. Drugs such as beta-blockers, clonidine, and ergotamines, which also cause vasoconstriction and could induce or aggravate Raynaud's disease, should be avoided. Raynaud's disease is associated with vibrating tools, so it is also sometimes called "vibration syndrome" or white finger, because the fingers turn pale.

Associated Disorders

Your doctor should be on the lookout for other disorders that may accompany, result from, be mistaken for, or complicate RSI.

Reflex Sympathetic Dysfunction (RSD)

Reflex sympathetic dysfunction (sometimes referred to as reflex sympathetic dystrophy, a later stage of the disease) is a complex chronic pain disorder affecting the sympathetic nervous system that can arise if RSI or other conditions are not treated properly. In RSD, pain leads to more pain, causing the person to avoid using the affected part, which perpetuates the pain cycle. The hallmark of RSD is severe, constant pain. It is frequently mistaken for thoracic outlet syndrome, carpal tunnel syndrome, rotator cuff injury, and cubital tunnel syndrome. Surgery for the last three can aggravate RSD.

Bone scan and other tests of the sensory, autonomic (involuntary), and motor aspect of the peripheral nervous system help confirm the clinical diagnosis.

In early stages, RSD causes burning pain. Later, vasoconstriction (reduced blood flow, usually characterized by coldness), weakness, tremors, spasms, and involuntary movements appear. People with RSD have trouble initiating movements (their hands don't "do as they are told"). In advanced stages, the skin is mottled, shiny, blue, or pale. Atrophy, loss of calcium, and serious depression can also occur.

Reflex sympathetic dysfunction can be worsened by treatments such as splints, bed rest, and ice massage; alcohol, barbiturates, drugs such as Valium, Librium, and Halcion; and foods containing nitrites and MSG, chocolate, red meat, and sharp cheese, so they should be avoided. In addition, surgery or injection can cause or worsen RSD. The best treatment is early, aggressive physical therapy, because it counteracts harmful immobility. Trigger point injections help ease pain and keep the area mobile. Massage, moist heat, and soaking in salt water helps. In later stages, sympathetic nerve ganglion blocks, beta-blockers or calcium channel blockers, and antidepressants are used.

Reflex sympathetic dysfunction must be diagnosed and treated within approximately six months of onset or it is likely to worsen and become chronic. Your physician must be skilled at making this diagnosis in order to catch it in time. People with RSD usually need psychotherapy to help deal with the pain.

Focal Dystonia (Writer's Cramp)

Focal dystonia, also known as writer's or occupational cramp, is an involuntary cramping of the hand that occurs because of misfired signals from the brain. Focal dystonia can be terrifying to people who have it. This condition can grow progressively worse without intervention.

Focal dystonia was described by Bernardino Ramazzini, the father of occupational medicine, who devoted a chapter to this "disease of scribes" in his book, *Disease of Workers*, published in 1713. He claimed scribes developed this writer's cramp from the "incessant driving of pen over paper." In 1888, W. R. Gowers also noted that the writer could not help holding his pen too tightly. Dr. Gowers wisely observed that this disease could be prevented if people would only write from their shoulders.

Though this condition is rare among computer workers, your doctor should ask if you have trouble with your handwriting, or find yourself making involuntary movements with your fingers. One woman described an experience common to people afflicted with focal dystonia: "If you look at checks I wrote five years ago with checks I write now, you'd see the difference in my handwriting. It's jerky. The O's aren't round; they come to a point. The slant goes different ways. My writing just deteriorates after a while. I can't keep letters equal."

Focal dystonia is a serious condition that needs to be treated early. There is no cure yet, but some cases are managed by serial injections of botulinum toxin and technique retraining. People who write a lot or use a stylus for the computer must be trained to hold it lightly and move the hand, as Dr. Gowers suggested, from the shoulder joint.

Degenerative Joint Disease (Osteoarthritis)

The question of whether degenerative joint disease (osteoarthritis) is a true repetitive strain injury is controversial; however, it compounds the problems of RSI. It affects both sexes, and by age 40 most people have some degree of this disease. Symptoms include morning stiffness, pain that is worsened by exercise, diminished range of motion in the joints, and cracking or grating sensations.

Exercise is the best way to prevent arthritis from worsening and to maintain healthy soft tissue. Aspirin and nonsteroidal anti-inflammatories are prescribed for pain.

Fibromyalgia

Though not a form of RSI, fibromyalgia, a controversial chronic pain disorder, has many symptoms that mimic RSI. The main hallmarks of fibromyalgia are painful "trigger points" at key sites of the body, and it involves aching, stiffness, or swelling in the neck, shoulders, back, and pelvis. Many people with this diagnosis say their sleep doesn't refresh them, and they wake up tired, aching, and stiff. Cold, humidity, and stress worsen symptoms, and heat, mild activity, and rest relieve them.

Fibromyalgia is treated with low-dose antidepressants to help regulate sleep, but nonsteroidal anti-inflammatories and other painkillers rarely help much. Aerobic exercise and stretching often help.

Dupuytren's Contracture

Dupuytren's disease, which begins with thickening of the palm or a nodule that first appears on the fascia attached to the tendon, sometimes leads to its characteristic contracture, with the finger pulling toward the palm. It usually affects the ring finger but can later affect the middle and little digits. Dupuytren's disease is more common among men than women, usually

THE CONTINUUM OF RSI

	Pre-RSI	Early RSI	Danger Zone	Chronic Pain	Complex Chronic Pain; Reflex Sympathetic Dysfunction
Symptom	"Funny" feeling in arms or hands.	Intermittent twinges of pain or tingling while typing.	Weakness, clumsiness; pain intermittent but not necessarily relieved by rest; daily activities impaired; depression.	Weakness, constant pain, not relieved by rest; made worse by any activity, disability.	Chronic pain; RSD, dystonia; severe depression.
Outcome	Relieved by rest.	Relieved by rest and rehabilitation.	Moderate risk of permanent impairment.	High risk of permanent impairment.	Permanent disability.

occurs after middle age, and can run in families. Whether Dupuytren's disease is caused by work is disputed, but it can certainly be aggravated if you type a lot, because the extensor tendons and muscles have to strain against the contracted tendon in the palm of the hand.

In cases where Dupuytren's disease has been treated surgically, occasionally complications, including reflex sympathetic dysfunction (described on page 58), can result. Unfortunately, at present, nonoperative techniques are considered ineffectual.

Don't Diagnose Yourself

Symptoms can mean many things. Don't drive yourself crazy with attempts at self-diagnosis if you experience some of the signs described above; see a qualified physician and get a medical opinion. Remember, if you aren't convinced your doctor is well versed in the complexities of RSI—or at least willing to investigate them with you—you can see another doctor. If you belong to a health maintenance organization, insist on getting a second opinion from a specialist.

Don't Panic

RSI develops over months and years, but when it finally settles in and doesn't go away even when computer use is discontinued, people tend to panic. Reading through a list of symptoms, and discovering their implications, can be frightening. Try to avoid thinking the worst while you wait for your appointment. It may not be as bad as you think; and in any case, worrying yourself to pieces won't help. What *will* help is to follow the retraining techniques described in Chapter 16. If you are still able to work, use the pacing technique described on page 185.

CHAPTER 7

The RSI Examination

A proper examination for repetitive strain injury should include a detailed history of your past and present general health and your current symptoms. Your muscles and nerves should be thoroughly tested for weakness or damage. Finally, your workstation and typing style should be analyzed for flaws that may have led to injury. This labor-intensive evaluation can take 60 to 90 minutes, but it is the only way to get a clear picture of the situation.

MEDICAL HISTORY

Your medical history provides a map for proper diagnosis, and your doctor should ask a lot of specific questions. All questions pertinent to the RSI examination can't be included here, but the following sampling—along with the explanations of why they are asked—should help you decide whether your physician is doing a thorough job.

How is your general health?

This tells the doctor whether there are any underlying problems that could complicate RSI, such as hypothyroidism, diabetes, arthritis, Lyme disease, or heart problems.

Have you seen any other health-care professionals about this problem?

Generally, people have been to five or six doctors or alternative health-care practitioners by the time they come to my office. It is useful to know other physicians' diagnoses and how this condition has been treated in the past. For instance, if a patient has already had surgery or been injected with steroids—which can damage muscle and tendon if used injudiciously—it can affect current treatment.

Have you ever injured your hands? Any change in the appearance of your hands?

Previous injuries, and how they were treated, can create weaknesses. Atrophy, swelling, or growths can indicate certain problems.

Do you sleep well?

Stress and fatigue contribute to RSI because tired muscles are more prone to injury; therefore, it is important to know whether a patient gets adequate rest. Insomnia can also occur with fibromyalgia, depression, and anxiety.

Do you smoke or drink?

Smoking and drinking can be indicative of a high-stress lifestyle; they also can make matters worse if you have RSI. See pages 38–39 for the risks associated with drinking and smoking.

How much time do you spend at the computer?

Computer jobs can be divided into four general categories by intensity of computer use:

Straight Input or Editing. Word processors, airlines reservation clerks, emergency dispatchers, directory assistance operators, and other people who type from prepared copy or verbal instructions for the entire workday are especially at risk because they can spend up to eight hours a day typing.

Intellectual Use. These occupations require people to compose at a computer, such as computer programming, journalism, and finance. If you have one of these jobs, you have built-in pauses because you alternate between thinking and typing. It is sometimes hard for people to gauge how much time they spend typing, but because they are absorbed in thought they may not realize how many hours they actually work. Just holding your hands to the keyboard and looking at the screen for long periods of time is stressful to the body, because static loading is injurious, too.

Mixed Use. People who have mixed job functions generally take information over the telephone, handwrite, and use a computer. Here all the job activities must be evaluated, and it may be difficult to figure out the time actually spent typing as opposed to holding the body in rigid postures. This kind of job is preferable to nonstop computer use, but if the person doing it types with the phone squeezed to his ear and shoulder, grips his pen, or rarely takes breaks, it can lead to injury.

Binge Work. Binge workers typically do not use the computer heavily on a daily basis, but when a big project comes along, their computer use increases dramatically. These people may go for days without using a computer, then spend 18 hours working on a big document. Jobs affected by seasonal peaks of activity, such as filing quarterly reports, probably involve binges of overwork at the computer.

If you spend over four hours at the keyboard during the course of the day, you have entered the danger zone for RSI.

Did you learn to type on a regular typewriter or a computer?
Did you have any trouble while using a typewriter? NO

People who learned to type on a typewriter may have had a formal typing class where they learned to keep their wrists straight. If you were able to use a regular typewriter without any problem, but started experiencing symptoms right after converting to a new kind of keyboard, then the trouble may have something to do with the keyboard.

Do you hunt and peck or touch-type?

Self-taught typists generally, but not always, have fewer problems because they don't ulnar deviate or rest their wrists while they hunt and peck.

How long have you worked at a computer? 5 YRS

Repetitive strain injury can take years to develop, so the doctor needs to know how long you've been working with computers and how many years you used a typewriter before that.

What kind of work do you do?

If you work with a mouse, or use the number pad almost exclusively, your dominant hand will bear the most stress.

Are you on the phone a lot?

If you type while you talk on the phone and don't use a headset, the doctor should look for neck problems.

Is your work machine-paced or can you go at your own speed?

Machine-paced work means a human being is expected to keep up with the computer, not vice versa. If your work allows for self-pacing while you stop and think, you are better off because you can take breaks. A person whose keystrokes are being counted, and who risks lowering productivity by going to the restroom for five minutes, has more problems during recovery.

What kind of keyboard do you use?

If you use a keyboard that has several rows of function keys, the inner muscles of your hands might be strained from improper technique.

Do you take breaks? If so, what is your idea of a break?

Patients often tell me work is so hectic they rarely leave their desks, much less get up and stretch. Stopping to drink coffee for 15 minutes every four hours or so is not enough. You need at least one 5- to 10-minute break for every 30 minutes at the computer, and one of those breaks should include stretching specific areas.

Not like this

Do you do any other heavy work with your hands?

Carpentry, gardening, playing a musical instrument, or even holding a steering wheel while driving could compound the computer-related trauma to your hands, so your doctor should ask about it. Some people use a home computer after working on one at the office all day and don't think to mention this extra usage unless they are prompted.

yes

Do you have young children?

A new baby can also put heavy stress on the hands, as anyone who has ever tried to hold a squirming infant in one arm while trying to do something else with the free hand can tell you. Hormonal changes caused by pregnancy can predispose you to carpal tunnel syndrome. These symptoms generally subside after giving birth.

No

(1) PLASTERING   (2) NECK

When did your problem begin and under what circumstances?

A reporter might answer, "When the war started and the stories came in faster than I could handle them." A computer operator might say that it corresponded with a particularly busy time during which she worked 12- to 18-hour days. Surges in workload can be the last straw for muscles that have struggled to keep up with the stress of computing.

Where does it hurt? Which hand is dominant?

Pain indicates where the doctor should start to look for the problem. It helps to know which hand is dominant, because if you are right-handed, and you work with the number pad all day, it tells the doctor that the workload is not being evenly distributed between two hands.

How are you presently coping with the problem? Are you able to do your job? Do your symptoms interfere with your daily activities?

The degree of pain you feel when you use a keyboard is an indication of the severity of your injury and helps the doctor to decide whether you should be allowed to work or whether your keyboard time should be curtailed. Can you still cut vegetables and push doors open? Or are you so affected you can't brush your teeth or comb your hair without triggering pain? If the activities of daily life are severely curtailed, using a keyboard may be out of the question.

Do you exercise? What kind of exercise do you do?

People who are in good physical shape are likely to do well in therapy, so if you exercise it tells the doctor that you are already taking good care of yourself and that you have a good head start. But although exercise is a good idea, there are certain kinds of exercise that can hurt you if you have RSI.

People who use computers need strength and flexibility in their upper body to meet the demands of computer work, so exercise routines designed to help you with that are taught in physical therapy. People who have a fitness program can continue with what they already do, or discuss safe modifications with an occupational therapist. People who don't have an exercise routine can find one they like; again, your rehabilitation therapist can be most helpful in that area.

Are you depressed or angry about this?

RSI can wreck careers, relationships, and self-esteem; it can lead to financial ruin and a host of difficulties. Needless to say, these pressures can create secondary psychological problems of rage, anxiety, and depression. You may need professional counseling to help you deal with these difficulties.

CLINICAL SIGNS OF RSI

After your doctor gets an idea of your history, the next step is a complete physical examination of the hand, wrist, forearm, shoulder, back, and neck. Your doctor will look for cysts, tumors, muscle atrophy, and swelling and apply gentle pressure to the forearms and hands to test for tenderness or swelling in muscles and joints. He will ask you to move your arms and shoulders in certain patterns to see if your range of motion is impaired and to notice the ease of motion with which you perform these tasks. Your posture, build, and muscle mass also need to be evaluated.

Because you will be doing a fair amount of squeezing and resistance during your examination, don't be surprised if you feel sore the next day. If you find the testing excruciating, though, tell your doctor. He can do more muscle testing when you're feeling less tender.

Hypermobility (Double-jointedness)

Hypermobility of the joints (double-jointedness) is a very important risk factor for RSI. For example, if you bend the tip of your finger upward at the joint and it goes back more than 20 degrees, you are hypermobile. In my study of injured computer operators, nearly three-quarters of them had one or more hypermobile finger or thumb joints. Unstable joints predispose you to injury because your muscles have to work extra hard to keep them positioned.

Muscle Damage

Muscle damage can cause problems other than biomechanical inefficiency. Muscles deteriorate and rebuild as a natural process of life, but when they are overused, the body can't catch up with the destruction of delicate tissues and may replace them with scar tissue, which is inelastic.

Overuse of the muscles causes cells to break down, releasing waste products, which produces pain and inflammation. Cleanup crews in the form of macrophages come to carry away the cellular debris. If you take anti-inflammatory drugs (such as aspirin) at this time, the natural inflammation process is disrupted, and instead of being cleansed away in the bloodstream, the trash settles into scar tissue. This scar tissue can bind muscles and tendons together, forcing them to work when they shouldn't have to. When someone has too much scar tissue, the risk of permanent disability looms large.

The Chain Reaction of Damage

Muscle shortening in the forearms also strains the tendons of the fingers because they have to work harder than they should. Tendons stretch very little, so the shortened muscle and tight tendon cause increased friction from shearing and you get further inflammation and tendinitis. Inflammation can cause swelling, which can make the tissue press on the nerve, and this can lead to neurological problems.

Testing Muscles

Wrist Flexion Test

Every muscle has an optimal length. Injury to muscles and the surrounding fascia and other soft tissue can cause them to shorten, and they become less efficient because they are out of balance: One side is too long, and the other is too short.

Forearm muscle shortening—a cardinal sign of RSI—frequently goes unrecognized by physicians. The normal wrist should be able to bend and flex to 70 to 90 degrees, but 90% of my RSI patients have impaired wrist flexion and extension, and some can barely bend their wrists in either direction because of muscle tightness.

Grip Strength

Weakness is one of the first signs of damage to the soft tissue, but most people have no idea that they are weak and are very surprised to discover it during an examination. To see how strong your grip is, your doctor may ask you to squeeze an instrument called a Jamar dynamometer, which measures the number of pounds you can pull. Your grip strength will be tested periodically during recovery as a way of measuring how much strength you've regained in your hands, which is a sign of recovery.

Pulp Pinch

The pulp pinch test measures the strength in your fingers. You'll be asked to squeeze the meter as hard as you can in different positions, such as pinching your thumb and forefinger together, or as if you were holding a door key.

Finkelstein's Sign

In the test for Finkelstein's sign, you will be asked to make a fist with the thumb curled inside. Then your doctor will bend your hand down and ask you if it hurts. This test can indicate deQuervain's disease.

TESTS FOR NERVE DAMAGE

Phalen's Maneuver

Your doctor will ask you to hold the backs of your hands together with your fingers facing the floor in a kind of upside-down prayer position for a minute or so. The purpose of this test is to see whether your fingers go numb or get tingly. A positive Phalen's test is one of several tests that confirm a diagnosis of carpal tunnel syndrome.

Tinel's Sign

Your doctor will tap with his finger on various anatomical sites, such as the elbow or the palm side of your wrist, to see if you feel any tingling. If you do, it is possible you have nerve irritation or compression.

Nerve Conduction Studies/Electromyography (EMG)

If you have a positive Phalen's or Tinel's test, your doctor may want you to have an electromyogram (EMG). An EMG consists of two parts to test motor and sensory nerves: nerve conduction studies and the needle EMG. The EMG machine has a monitor that shows what happens in the body when a low voltage of electricity passes through specified areas.

Before beginning, the doctor or lab technician will wrap a cuff around your wrist that acts as a ground wire for safety. In the first part of the test, the doctor will tape two electrodes a little smaller than a dime to your finger and palm. Then she will hold a stimulation bar a few measured inches away and, with a tap to a foot pedal, send about five separate pulses of progressively stronger electrical current through the wires, which feels like a mild electric shock. The EMG machine records the impulses, and the doctor averages the five samples to minimize the effect of static. This reading allows the doctor to detect signs of nerve damage.

Testing is repeated along various sites of the arm to see where nerve damage might have occurred. Later, two coil rings are placed on your fingers instead of the electrode discs.

The second part of the test, the needle EMG, records normal electrical activity within the muscle. Here, the doctor will tape an electrode about the size of a half-dollar to the top of your wrist and insert a needle shallowly along certain muscles. The needles will be inserted at various sites along the arm, such as the web of your thumb and forefinger, your biceps, your forearms, and other places, depending on your symptoms. Your doctor will ask you to exert force in certain directions, for instance, to pull your arm up while your doctor is holding it down, and the activity is recorded on the EMG. This allows your doctor to detect signs of nerve damage.

The amount of pain you feel during an EMG will depend on your sensitivity to pain. It helps to try to relax; anxiety can worsen the pain.

The nerve conduction velocity study is considered the gold standard for verifying carpal tunnel syndrome. However, there can be borderline findings, so it is best to take the entire clinical examination into account before opting for surgery.

NOTE: Moisturizers or other creams can interfere with proper testing, so don't apply any to your arm from the time of your last shower to your appointment. Cold hands can also impede testing, so your doctor may have you warm them with hot water.

Semmes-Weinstein Monofilament Test

The Semmes-Weinstein monofilament test is a cheap, easy, and painless way to see whether or not you have lost the ability to feel light touch in your hands. This fine sensitivity helps protect you from burning yourself, for instance. The instrument used in the test looks rather like a toothbrush with one long bristle, and your doctor will ask you to close your eyes and say "yes" if you feel anything while he touches parts of your fingertips, palm, and wrist with the filament. If you can't feel anything, you may have suffered nerve damage and your doctor may order a nerve conduction/ electromyogram (EMG) to verify this.

The Weber Two-Point Discrimination Test

The Weber two-point discrimination test also tests light-touch sensibility using an instrument that looks like a pizza wheel with irregularly placed spokes. The doctor will ask you to close your eyes and say whether you feel one or two points when she touches your fingertips with the blunt wire prongs. The closer the interval, the harder it will be to discriminate between one and two points.

Magnetic Resonance Imaging (MRI)

Magnetic resonance imaging allows a doctor to see through skin, muscle, and bone. In this noninvasive, painless (but sometimes claustrophobia-producing) procedure, a scanner moves along the body, which is placed within a magnetic field, taking "pictures" as it goes along.

An MRI helps your doctor assess whether there is a tear or inflammation of soft tissue, most often in the shoulder, which contains many muscles, tendons, ligaments, and lubricant sacs (bursae).

X Rays

Damage to the soft tissue doesn't usually show up on plain X rays. However, if your doctor suspects a bone or joint problem or arthritis, an X ray may be in order.

VIDEO ANALYSIS

During the final, and perhaps most crucial, part of the examination, patients are videotaped at a simulated workstation. Videotape is an invaluable tool, because people can see exactly what they are doing to provoke injury. I tape two examples: one of the way they usually work, and then one of how they look when they use proper technique. That way, they can compare the before and after versions. Invariably, there is a moment of "Aha!" understanding (usually accompanied by a relieved grin) when RSI patients link awkward positions with their pain by seeing themselves in action.

Videotape is also an effective persuader: People rarely believe me when I tell them what they are doing, but the camera doesn't lie. It is also difficult for people to understand what good positioning means, but seeing it on the screen makes it easier to grasp. A practiced eye is required to see the tiny movement that can be so damaging when repeated over and over during the course of a day. One example is the rapid typist who quickly ulnar deviates to reach the Caps Lock key. It happens in an instant—instead of moving the whole hand, the little finger stretches to the side. With a video camera, the action can be stopped and the person can see the strain in his or her hands on the screen.

First, I ask people to set up the chair, keyboard, and copyholder to approximate what they have at work. Then I videotape them typing, using the number pad or function keys that they typically use at work, until I get a good sample of their style. Then I replay the tape and show them which positions and habits are causing problems. Last, I readjust the workstation to fit them, and I show them safe ways to hold their hands. Then I make another film so they can see how relaxed and unstressed their hands look by comparison. (For details on this essential retraining, see Chapter 16.)

If your doctor doesn't have a video camera and simulated workstation, have a friend videotape you (ideally, you should be taped at your actual workstation). If this isn't possible, have someone take pictures of you working at your desk. The photographs should include aerial and profile views. This won't be as good as a videotape, but it will give your doctor an idea of your ergonomic situation and your typical posture.

CHAPTER 8

Treatment Options for RSI

Before you start considering treatment options for RSI, your physician must first determine the extent of your injury. People with moderate to mild injuries may be able to continue working through recovery, as long as they modify their workstations, learn how to position their hands properly, and undergo physical therapy. Severely injured people may need many months to a year or more off work to recuperate. Some people will never be able to work at a keyboard again.

A slow, conservative approach generally brings the best results.

THE ROLE OF REST

Muscles heal better when they are allowed to move, because that way the newly grown tissue remains pliable. So the term *rest* (in the sense of taking to your bed) is misleading in this context. When people lie in bed and do nothing, their muscles contract. With RSI, the contraction process has already begun because damaged muscles hurt and shrink, which creates a vicious cycle of pain and contraction. Rest means that you should not do anything to stress the injured muscles, so you should refrain from doing (or overdoing) activities that led to RSI (such as using the computer) or that exacerbate your symptoms (such as knitting, playing musical instruments, gardening, or carpentry).

The rest period is also the time you'll undergo aggressive physical therapy—receiving deep tissue massage once to three times a week. During your diagnosis, you learned which muscle groups needed to be stretched and strengthened. Now your physical therapist will teach you how to perform stretching and strengthening exercises, gradually adding new exercises, weights, and elastic exercise bands (stretchy strips of latex that are used in exercise routines) as you progress. You will do these exercises at home every day. You should also ask your physical therapist any questions you have about your injury. The therapist can offer valuable suggestions, so take advantage of this opportunity.

SPLINTING

To understand splinting, you must first understand how tissue heals. When soft tissue tears, scarring occurs. This scar tissue grows randomly at the site of injury and must be encouraged to grow in the right direction (and prevented from adhering to the wrong place, such as bones) by gentle movement. So immobility can prolong, or make chronic, an injury that would have healed if the normal movement were allowed. People usually view pain as a signal that they are harming themselves, but this isn't necessarily so in soft tissue injury. Though this theory is perfectly logical and sometimes correct, in soft tissue injury certain gentle movements are necessary for proper healing.

To Splint or Not to Splint

Whether the injury is properly treated by rest or movement depends on the diagnosis. If a mobile scar is needed, as in the case of a soft tissue injury, you need to keep moving. If a firm scar is necessary, as in the case of a broken bone, you need to immobilize the area with a splint or cast. Sometimes a part-time splint is appropriate.

Unfortunately, too many doctors and physical therapists treat soft tissue injuries with unnecessary splints, prolonging the damage and setting the stage for chronic injuries that could otherwise have healed. Some people splint themselves in a misguided attempt to "prevent" RSI, which can be injurious in itself as well as aggravate existing injuries. Splints are advertised in catalogs to "prevent" RSI, and some people use splints without medical supervision "to keep their wrists straight" when they type. This is something you should learn to do on your own. It is particularly dangerous to type with a splint on, because over time it can cause atrophy in one group of muscles and overuse in another, and atrophy happens fast. You can lose a significant amount of your muscle power within two weeks.

Using splints inappropriately also can cause RSI symptoms to migrate. Splints restrict motion, so you make postural compromises and strain another part of your anatomy. They can also lead to deformities of the tissues or reflex sympathetic dystrophy. I've seen some real disasters caused by splints. Better not to splint unless absolutely necessary, and get rid of the splint as soon as possible. Never splint yourself—ask your doctor if you really need one.

The Proper Use of Splints

Splints should be prescribed by your physician for specific problems, such as deQuervain's disease or carpal tunnel syndrome, on a limited basis. If splints are used for carpal tunnel syndrome, they should be worn only at night, unless your physician tells you otherwise. Splints are worn at night to prevent people from flexing their wrists in their sleep. (If you're wearing them for deQuervain's disease to prevent thumb movement, they may be worn in the daytime, but only if you are not typing.) Make sure you understand the purpose for your splint completely before you leave the doctor's office.

Addicted to Splints

Splints alleviate the pain somewhat, so people get hooked on them. This problem could be avoided entirely if there were more effort placed on stretching and strengthening the muscles. If you are addicted to splints, try weaning yourself from them by using them for one hour on, then one hour off, then one hour on, then two hours off, gradually increasing the time off until you are free of them completely.

Mental Splinting

Rather than relying on a crutch, learn to let your own muscles support you. One patient described knowing the correct position of her arms as "mental splinting." This is an excellent concept: She was describing using her own musculature to keep her bones in proper alignment, something everyone should do. This is not meant to imply that rigidity is okay, however.

DRUG TREATMENT

Nonsteroidal Anti-inflammatory Analgesics

Nonsteroidal anti-inflammatory drugs (NSAIDs) are commonly prescribed for the pain and inflammation caused by RSI, but they have several side effects and limited usefulness. Some doctors have given up prescribing them for RSI, feeling that NSAIDS don't work and in fact interfere with the body's natural attempt to clear the bloodstream of debris that will form scar tissue. Ice is effective in controlling pain, and it reduces inflammation without interfering with this important cleansing process. Vitamin E, an antioxidant, also shows promise in this area (see page 81).

Commonly prescribed NSAIDs include drugs containing ibuprofen (such as Advil, Nuprin, Motrin, Anaprox, and Tolectin) or fenoprofen (such as Nalfon). More potent and less commonly prescribed NSAIDs are Butazolidin, Indocin, and Voltaren. Side effects can be serious, especially for people over 40. There are dozens of possible side effects: ulcers or bleeding, stomach cramps, nausea or indigestion, chills, fluid retention, kidney impairment, fever or other flu-like symptoms, headache, insomnia, and sun sensitivity, to name a few.

Anti-inflammatories can infrequently cause a severe allergic reaction known as anaphylaxis, which requires immediate medical attention. According to the *United States Pharmacopeia Complete Drug Reference*, danger signs include very fast or irregular breathing, gasping for breath, fainting, hivelike swellings of the skin, and fast but irregular heartbeat or pulse. If this happens, you should ask someone to drive you to the nearest hospital emergency room. "If this is not possible, do not try to drive yourself. Call an ambulance, lie down, cover yourself to keep warm, and prop your feet higher than your head. Stay in that position until help arrives."

Be sure to tell your doctor about any side effects to the drug. Your doctor should also know if you have a history of alcohol or tobacco use, bleeding problems, ulcers, diabetes, hepatitis, heart disease, asthma, or high blood pressure if you are going to use NSAIDs.

If you take NSAIDs, take the pills with food or an antacid. Antacids containing magnesium and aluminum hydroxides are recommended by the *Pharmacopeia*, which has a detailed section on this medication that is well worth reading. Your pharmacist can also answer questions about proper use of these drugs.

Aspirin

Aspirin is also used to treat the pain of RSI. As ubiquitous as aspirin taking is, and as generally safe as aspirin is considered to be, you should still treat it with the same kind of respect due any drug. Aspirin can interact with alcohol and other drugs and may cause side effects. People with liver or kidney disease, peptic ulcer, or bleeding problems may not be able to take aspirin. You should never take aspirin if you are taking an NSAID unless your doctor tells you to do so and is monitoring your progress.

Acetaminophen

Acetaminophen is an aspirin substitute for pain control that elevates the pain threshold but is unlikely to produce the side effects of aspirin. It is sold under the name of Tylenol, among others. It should not be taken with aspirin, Voltaren, Nalfon, or certain other drugs for more than a few days, unless your doctor tells you to do so and is monitoring your progress.

Cortisone Injections

Injections of cortisone are used to treat RSI, but they should be used sparingly, if at all. Cortisone is very strong medicine, and such injections are disliked in some medical circles because the drug can cause tendons to rupture. People who have these injections frequently don't do as well. It is not uncommon to hear patients say, "Everything's fine *except* the place where they injected cortisone." I do not use this treatment; however, some physicians believe that cortisone injections can sometimes be helpful in reducing pain and inflammation when carefully adminstered by an experienced, competent physician.

Cortisone should not be injected into unstable joints, and you should not overuse the affected area as long as you are having symptoms. Cortisone may produce systemic as well as local effects, such as fluid retention, and it can cause allergic reactions, muscle weakness, and loss of muscle mass. If you experience any side effects from cortisone injections, call your physician.

Cortisone Creams and Sprays

In addition to injection, cortisone can also be applied in other ways, such as in creams and sprays. Some physical therapists apply creams containing a 10% cortisone solution on fibrous tissue and rub an ultrasound or electrical device over the cream. These processes, called phonophoresis and iontophoresis, respectively, allow the cortisone to penetrate through the skin to the tissue to reduce inflammation.

SURGERY

During a lecture on RSI, Dr. Robert Markison, a hand surgeon and associate clinical professor of surgery at the University of California, San Francisco, remarked that a dangerous situation arises when vulnerable patients fall into the hands of unscrupulous surgeons. "The doctor says, 'You need carpal tunnel surgery. I've got a knife. I've got time.'" Rather than being "passive dependent consumers of medicine," as Dr. Markison put it, arm yourself with knowledge about what the procedure entails, and get a second opinion before you have surgery. A good surgeon will not operate unless it is necessary. Markison noted that his most trusted surgeon friends are equally happy with aspects of treatment that do not involve operations. "We delight in nonsurgical treatments," he said.

The first thing to be aware of regarding surgery and RSI is that in most cases, the damage to muscle and tendon cannot be surgically repaired. If this tissue heals at all, it will happen slowly, through rest and physical therapy. Surgical procedures do exist for carpal tunnel syndrome, Dupuytren's contracture, deQuervain's disease, ulnar nerve entrapment, and several other afflictions mentioned in this book.

Weighing Your Options

Surgery is sometimes necessary to preserve nerve function, without which you could lose protective sensation in the hands, or to prevent the pressure caused by the bone overgrowth of osteoarthritis from crowding the median nerve. However, surgery has been implicated in the onset of reflex sympathetic dysfunction, especially with carpal tunnel syndrome and Dupuytren's contracture, so it is not something to be taken lightly.

Getting a Second Opinion

It is always wise to get a second opinion before having surgery. Treatment for carpal tunnel syndrome—and many other conditions—is not a one-way street. It doesn't have to lead to surgery.

Some people feel pressured by their employers to have the surgery in the mistaken notion that this will "cure" the problem and allow the employee to return to work. If an employee refuses to have surgery, sometimes the Workers' Compensation representative accuses the employee of not wanting to get better, which creates an unfortunate catch-22.

Be sure that surgery is really necessary before you agree to it, because it is serious and can lead to poor results, as described earlier. On the other hand, if your doctor (or doctors, if you get a second opinion) gives you a good reason for surgery, then you should consider it.

Carpal Tunnel Surgery

Carpal tunnel surgery is a relatively simple procedure. The surgeon cuts the transverse carpal ligament to create more room in the carpal tunnel. By doing this, the pressure on the median nerve is released, so you don't have numbness and tingling or risk atrophy of the thumb muscle. For advanced cases, where the lining of the nerve—the epineurium—has thickened, the surgeon removes scar tissues from the nerve and its lining.

You may need surgery if your pain is intolerable, or if your thumb muscle starts to atrophy. There is a window of time—about a year to a year and a half—after which you run the risk of permanent nerve damage. Generally, four to six weeks must elapse before you can use your hands in daily work after such surgery.

Endoscopic (Keyhole) Surgery. Traditional carpal tunnel release surgery leaves a scar on the palm of the hand, and sometimes people experience burning over the scar tissue or chronic wrist pain afterward. A new technique using fiberoptic tools allows the surgeon to make a smaller incision.

Recovery time from this surgery is half the time required by traditional surgery.

Some surgeons hail endoscopic surgery as the wave of the future; others say they prefer the traditional release because they can see more that way than through the endoscope, which the surgeon must view on a television monitor rather than firsthand.

A new surgical technique similar to balloon angioplasty for the heart is also being used. The surgeon makes a small incision at the base of the palm and inflates a balloon under the ligament, which stretches the ligament— rather than cutting it—to free the pressure on the nerve.

Ulnar Nerve Transposition. If your ulnar nerve lies close to the surface, the nerve can be easily damaged by leaning on your elbow, or the friction caused by flexing and stretching your forearm, as in sulcus ulnaris syndrome or cubital tunnel syndrome. Surgery to correct this involves moving the ulnar nerve to another location and then burying it in muscle or fat to protect it from irritation.

Surgery for DeQuervain's Disease. Surgery for deQuervain's disease or other tendon entrapments is usually done on an outpatient basis, using local anesthesia. It takes two to eight weeks to heal from this operation. Because human anatomy varies, and there can be subtunnels with the deQuervain's tunnel needing separate release, this surgery should be done by an experienced surgeon.

ALTERNATIVE TREATMENTS

A study published in the *New England Journal of Medicine* found that an estimated 34% of Americans used alternative therapy in 1990; and 72% of them did not tell their doctors about it, which suggests a deficiency in current patient-doctor relations.

People seek alternative therapies for a number of reasons: They dislike taking powerful drugs with adverse side effects, and would rather try more benign treatments; they perceive that their doctor doesn't listen to them or doesn't care about their problem, whereas their holistic practitioner does; and alternative therapies are cheaper than visits to the doctor.

Because people frequently seek alternative treatments with RSI, a few are discussed here. I do not necessarily advocate them, but if they help you feel better and do not hurt you, there is no harm in using them *provided* you use them under the guidance of your physician. Alternative therapies should not be used in the absence of a medical diagnosis. A team approach is far wiser.

Acupuncture

Because acupuncture stimulates the creation of beta-endorphins, the body's natural painkillers, it is sometimes highly effective in treating pain, and for that reason it may help certain RSI patients. In traditional Chinese acupuncture, fine needles are shallowly inserted along certain points located all over the body (the points often coincide with "trigger points," which when pressed will bring on pain) and left in place for approximately 20 to 40 minutes. Sometimes the points can feel tender, but acupuncture is not usually painful; it is certainly nothing like getting a shot or having blood drawn. Some acupuncturists use moxibustion, a technique in which a burning herb (usually mugwort) is held close to the needle for a few seconds. This can feel soothing and warming, but if it is not done carefully, it can cause burns and scarring.

If you seek acupuncture, be certain that your certified and licensed acupuncturist uses disposable needles. Some Western medical doctors are trained in acupuncture, so your treatment can be covered by insurance. Because it can be deeply relaxing, acupuncture is also useful for stress reduction, depression, and the anxiety caused by RSI.

Acupuncture should be used in conjunction with physical therapy and retraining, because you still need deep tissue massage to remodel scar tissue and technique retraining to prevent reinjury from poor technique.

Spinal Manipulation

Some patients find relief with hands-on manipulation performed by osteopathic doctors (who have equivalent training as M.D.'s) and chiropractors. This treatment can help to correct disturbances of the nervous, muscular, and vascular systems caused by improper alignment of the spine and limbs. However, sometimes manipulation makes joints so lax that they fall out of alignment, which can be a problem with RSI.

Vitamins

Antioxidants—vitamin C, vitamin E, and beta-carotene (yellow or red pigments found in carrot juice)—have been hailed for their possible role in fighting heart disease and cancer and preventing cataracts and hardening of the arteries. In addition to ensuring good bodily functioning, certain vitamins may be helpful in treating the problems created by RSI.

However, bear in mind that vitamins can't replace a good diet. A useful analogy was made by Jeffrey Blumberg, associate director of the USDA's Human Nutrition Research Center on Aging at Tufts University. "Vitamins are like seat belts," said Dr. Blumberg. "Wearing a seat belt doesn't give you a license to drive recklessly, it just protects you in case of an accident. Vitamin supplements work the same way: they won't give you a license to eat poorly and otherwise abuse your health, but provide an added cushion of protection."

Eat low on the food chain, with fresh fruits, vegetables, and whole grains making up the bulk of your diet. Think of meat, dairy products, fat, sugar, and oil as condiments. Remember, vitamins alone won't give you energy, and they certainly won't make up for poor dietary choices.

Also be aware that in large doses, vitamins are considered drugs and can have toxic effects on your body. Always talk to your doctor or nutritionist about the right dosage of any vitamin supplement you take so that it can be adjusted to your own needs.

Vitamin C. Vitamin C helps heal wounds, so be sure you are getting enough of it if you have RSI. Smokers, alcoholics, and people under prolonged stress may be deficient in vitamin C.

Vitamin E. According to a report in the *New York Times*, researchers at the Department of Agriculture's Human Nutrition Research Center on Aging at Tufts University found that vitamin E can minimize much of the muscle damage and inflammation that normally results from exercise. Oxygen radicals coursing through the muscle tissue can damage it by attacking the fats in cell membranes, leaving the membranes open to injury. The group who took 800 international units of vitamin E a day for a week before running downhill on a treadmill for 45 minutes produced fewer by-products of fat oxidation than a control group. "The vitamin also reduced blood levels of two chemical messengers that promote inflammation, which in turn should reduce post-exercise inflammation and soreness," according to the report.

So it may be worthwhile to take a vitamin E supplement for the soreness and inflammation of RSI. Vitamin E doesn't usually cause side effects,

---

Eat Your Vitamins

Vitamin A is found in fish liver oil, butter, cream, liver, and eggs. These are foods you should probably eat sparingly.

Vitamin C is found in citrus fruit, tomatoes, pepper, broccoli, potatoes, and cabbage.

Vitamin E is found in wheat germ, safflower and soybean oil, green leafy vegetables, legumes, and nuts.

Vitamin B$_6$ is found in meats, fish, legumes, egg yolks, peanuts, whole-grain cereals, bananas, and lima beans.

Beta-carotene is found in carrots, sweet potatoes, spinach, and yellow fruits.

according to the *Pharmacopeia*, but very large doses taken for a long time can cause blurred vision, diarrhea, dizziness, headache, nausea, or unusual weakness or fatigue.

Vitamin B$_6$. Vitamin B$_6$ (pyridoxine) is necessary for the proper functioning of the nervous system and blood cells. This vitamin is found in bananas, egg yolks, and whole-grain cereals, among other foods. The use of vitamin B$_6$ to diminish the pain of carpal tunnel syndrome is controversial, so check with your doctor before taking it.

Bodywork and Massage

Many people find that bodywork therapy helps them keep their muscles stretched or cope with stress. There are a number of different bodywork therapies: some kinds of bodywork, such as Rolfing and Hellerwork, involve deep tissue manipulation; others such as the Alexander or Feldenkrais Technique stress proper movement and alignment. Yoga also helps keep muscles stretched, and some postures, such as the twist or the eye exercises, seem tailor-made for RSI patients. (Some other postures, such as the Handstand, Frog, and Plough, however, should be avoided by people with RSI until and unless they have regained a lot of strength and flexibility because of the stress they put on the hands and neck.)

These postural retraining techniques may be quite helpful to you in continuing your home-care program and improving your postural awareness, especially after you stop physical therapy. It is also helpful to do these things in a group or class setting, so you have a coach to encourage you to do your best and not get lazy about postural alignment.

Massage therapy can also be wonderfully refreshing and can relieve pain and stress from computer work. Being massaged on a regular basis—and more frequently if you're under a lot of pressure or feel tight—can help keep your body supple and relaxed. Some people consider massage as much a part of their health regimen as is their workout.

Ask your physical or occupational therapist for suggestions of techniques that might help you continue your self-care program.

A Warning about Home Remedies

Many RSI patients are admirably motivated and will use homespun remedies in their attempt to speed healing. Please let your doctor know if you decide to buy a hand exerciser or home ultrasound device, or use other methods to treat yourself. It might be okay, *but it also might not be a good idea*, so check it out with your doctor first.

CHAPTER 9

Computer Vision

Is it possible to develop repetitive strain injury of the eye? James Sheedy, associate clinical chief of the VDT Eye Clinic at the University of California Berkeley School of Optometry, thinks it may be. According to Dr. Sheedy, nearsightedness and problems with the focusing mechanisms of the eye develop in computer workers. However, unlike some forms of RSI, many of these eye problems can be corrected.

In survey after survey, vision woes are among the most commonly cited complaints of computer users. According to the 1991 Steelcase Worldwide Office Environment Index by Louis Harris & Associates, Inc., 47% of the office workers polled named eyestrain as a serious health concern. One survey conducted by Dr. Sheedy found that 7 million patients went to their eye doctors for vision complaints related to video display terminals (VDTs) every year in the United States. According to a retrospective report concerning the patients in Dr. Sheedy's VDT eye clinic, 80% of the patients reported eyestrain and 50% reported blurred vision and headaches.

Eyestrain and headaches are the two most common complaints, but computer users also report neck and back pain, double or blurred vision, burning sensations, ocular fatigue, and other visual disturbances. So far, no lasting damage to an operator's vision has been conclusively attributed to computer design. However, this does not mean that good, comfortable vision isn't crucial to your well-being; it is.

In addition to making you comfortable at work, good vision helps reduce the risk of RSI by ensuring that you aren't making postural compromises to compensate for impaired eyesight—such as craning your neck or squinting to see your work or avoid glare from the screen.

Don't take fatigue and discomfort for granted. You should be able to see well and also sustain comfortable vision while working.

COMPUTER-RELATED EYE PROBLEMS

Computer use presents the eye with a number of unfamiliar tasks. Both the distance from the computer screen and its upright angle are an entirely new experience for the eye. And unlike a page from a book, computer monitors are both self-illuminating and reflective, so glare and reflection from overhead lights, windows, and bright white clothing can further burden vision.

Any sustained visual task, such as reading, can tax the eyes, but long, uninterrupted hours of staring at the computer screen tires the ocular focusing mechanism. It is possible to "charley horse" the eyes: Your eyes don't readjust to distance viewing and you are temporarily nearsighted. This can happen even if you wear corrective lenses.

Bifocals

Bifocal wearers have a built-in problem, because their prescriptions are designed for reading at a distance of approximately 16 inches, whereas the typical monitor is roughly 22 to 24 inches away from the eye. Bifocals are angled downward at 25 degrees for comfortable reading, but the optimal angle for viewing the computer screen is 10 to 15 degrees below horizontal. Bifocal wearers often thrust their necks into bad positions because they tilt their heads back to see the screen. If you wear bifocals and you get headaches when you work, this is a likely cause. Have your bifocals adjusted for computer work. Measure the distance from your eye to your monitor and give that information to your eye doctor.

Contact Lenses

The eyes of contact lens wearers can be irritated from computer work, too, because they blink less during deep periods of concentration. Dry eyes also result from improper humidity levels, a common problem in office buildings. If you wear contacts, remember to blink (program your computer to prompt you or put a sign where you can see it). It also helps to use artificial tears to reduce irritation—apply them as needed.

NOTE: Don't confuse artificial tears with products containing vasoconstrictors that remove redness from the eyes, which can mask symptoms you and your doctor should know about.

Avoiding Vision-Related Problems

Most people don't realize it, but testing for 20/20 vision is not adequate for computer work. It is quite possible to have other minor visual deficiencies—such as difficulties in the eye focusing mechanism or alignment—that you are unaware of until you're faced with the ocular challenges of VDT work. If you do, computer work can compound the eyestrain, neck pain, and headache that you experience from these hidden problems.

Have Your Vision Checked

To avoid problems, have your vision checked once a year by a competent eye doctor. Your optometrist or ophthalmologist should know precisely how you use your eyes on the job; test you for the work you are required to do; and design your prescription to make those tasks effortless. In fact, your eyes should be so comfortable that you are not even aware of them.

Before your appointment, measure the distance from your eyes to the monitor so your doctor can test your vision at that distance. Also tell your doctor how high the monitor sits on your desk, and whatever else needs to be clearly seen within your field of vision at work. Bring photos or a video of yourself working, if possible. According to Melvin Schrier, who treats many computer users in Manhattan, there are a number of skills your eye doctor should check:

- *Near-point visual acuity*—the ability to see clearly and efficiently at reading distance.
- *Binocularity*—the ability to fuse the image recorded by each eye into a single image.
- *Accommodation*—the ability of the eyes to shift focus between varying distances. (This affects operators who are over 40 years old, because the crystalline lens that allows for accommodation gradually becomes less flexible with age.)
- *Oculomotor skills*—the ability of the eye muscles to position the eyes correctly when locating and keep their place while reading or scanning text.

Schrier says that your doctor should also test for *hyperphoria*—the tendency of each eye to see objects at a different level. This is a very common—but rarely treated—disorder that forces people to tilt their heads in order to line things up visually. Hyperphoria can cause a great deal of neck strain.

You should be careful to set up your workstation properly. One of my patients was forced to sit at an angle to her monitor, and the constant strain of looking to the side made her eye muscle twitch, which could be called a sort of repetitive strain injury of the eye. See Chapter 15 for proper workstation setup.

Choose the Prescription that Works for You

No single prescription suits everyone. Some people like glasses, others prefer contact lenses. Some people get special glasses just for computer use. Others, such as bifocal wearers, have their glasses adjusted to both reading

---

VISION TIPS

- Rest your eyes for at least five minutes an hour. You can combine this with the stretch breaks (see page 184).

- During your rest periods, walk to a window and let your eyes rove over distant objects. Gaze at the leaves on a tree, follow a flock of birds with your eyes, or study the detailing of a faraway building. At the very least, focus on something across the room. See page 105 for eye exercises.

- Keep your screen clean. Dust can interfere with easy visibility.

---

and computer distances so they don't have to change glasses when they get up and walk around. Tell your doctor what you need and prefer, and work out the prescription that is right for you.

PART III

THE ROAD TO RECOVERY

CHAPTER 10

Beginning the Healing Process with Physical and Occupational Therapy

The art of medicine consists in amusing the patient while Nature cures the disease.

— Voltaire

In the traditional view of the doctor-patient relationship, people get sick and a doctor cures them. This lopsided perception puts the physician in the knowing, curative position and takes away all power—and responsibility—from the patient.

In real life, things are more complicated than that. Many ailments cannot be cured by a miracle drug—and the remedies for lifestyle-related conditions require strict patient compliance. Your doctor can tell you what you should eat, but he doesn't have any control over what you actually do.

Nowadays, people are much more informed about medicine than they used to be. Health magazines abound, and people read about the latest medical breakthroughs in the newspaper. This is good, because no doctor has the time to tell you every facet of a condition you might have. Being an informed medical consumer helps you be a better patient. Furthermore, if you don't inform yourself about your own condition you risk undergoing treatment you do not want. Informed patients, on the other hand, can knowledgeably discuss their options with their doctor and arrive at decisions on treatment together.

DOCTOR-PATIENT COLLABORATION

If you are diagnosed with RSI, try to view the doctor-patient relationship as a collaboration in which the doctor guides, advises, and aids in decisions regarding your treatment and you take charge of your recovery. Your doctor gives you a reliable diagnosis; then you help yourself by carefully following instructions. This could include resting, strengthening and stretching your muscles, and pacing yourself at work. The word *doctor* means teacher, which is the true function of a physician. This can be particularly true with RSI, if the doctor teaches patients how to take care of their injury through pain management, pacing, and technique retraining.

REHABILITATION THROUGH PHYSICAL AND OCCUPATIONAL THERAPY

People develop RSI because they don't know how to protect their muscles; the workstation was not set up correctly; they were never trained to use their hands properly; and they don't know how—or aren't allowed—to pace themselves. Add to this a lot of pressure or an unrealistically heavy workload.

To reverse the damage of RSI, these things need to change, and the process begins in rehabilitation therapy. You must learn to pace yourself in order to allow your muscles to rest. Pain-induced immobility is replaced by gentle stretching and strengthening exercises. Deep tissue massage breaks down scar tissue built up over years of overuse. Retraining arrests the cycle of reinjury. After doing all of this, you may still not heal as quickly as you would like, so try to be patient with yourself.

After your initial diagnosis, unless you have extremely mild RSI, you will probably enter occupational or physical therapy. The main difference between these specialties is emphasis: Both perform deep tissue massage, but physical therapists employ postural retraining, ultrasound, and other special treatments. Occupational therapists have special expertise in modifying splints and helping people with day-to-day activities, such as adapting sports equipment or the home environment. You can benefit from the expertise of either or both.

You'll probably wind up doing similar exercises in either case. Your therapist will use several techniques to help you get better, including application of heat and ice and deep tissue massage. Your therapist will also teach you exercises to do at home, advise you about pacing at work, and teach you the elements of good postural alignment. Take advantage of your therapist's expertise—therapists are full of good advice about how to help you and usually are very willing to dispense it.

Here are descriptions of several kinds of treatment. You might find some of them more effective than others. You may also benefit from a certain treatment more during one stage of recovery.

Heat Packs

Heat packs can relieve chronic pain, such as that of reflex sympathetic dysfunction, and are appropriate for long-term, rather than acute, injury. Your physical therapist may apply a heat pack before deep tissue massage to relax your muscles. This prepares the muscles for the remodeling of scar tissue.

Deep Tissue Massage

Injury to muscles causes them to shorten and become biomechanically inefficient. Inflammation causes scar tissue, which binds together muscles that should act independently, inhibiting their normal sliding action. Deep tissue massage, performed one to three times a week for several weeks or months by a rehabilitation therapist, will help reshape that scar tissue and reverse the process, allowing the muscle to heal. The therapist uses a long, stroking action that goes deep into the muscle and tendon, so it won't feel like other kinds of massage, such as Swedish or shiatsu.

Unfortunately, you can't massage yourself this way if your RSI affects both sides because you would strain your hands. In addition, you can't relax the way you could if someone else were doing the massaging. Some patients ask if a friend or spouse can give them massages. Talk to your physical or occupational therapist and doctor about that; they may be able to teach that person how to help you at home.

People experience pain differently, so pressure that feels good to one patient may be excruciating to another. Deep tissue massage should "hurt good"—that is, it should feel "right" even if it is mildly painful. But you should not find physical therapy agonizing; that is counterproductive, because you'll be tensing your muscles against expected pain instead of relaxing them. Tell your physical therapist if something is too painful.

NOTE: Because this therapy goes quite deep, you might feel sore or bruised after deep tissue massage. This is generally harmless and will heal.

Maintenance Massage

You probably won't be in physical therapy for the rest of your life, but if you keep typing, you're bound to build up strain and tension, even with the best self-care. Some medical insurance will cover massage if your doctor writes a note for you. It would be nice if everyone could get maintenance-level physical therapy to keep people in optimum shape, but that is not the case at present.

However, I highly recommend that you find a good massage therapist to work on your arms, neck, hands, and shoulders after you leave physical therapy to deal with residual stress, even if you must pay for it yourself. If you can afford to see someone once a week, that would be great. If you don't have the money to pay someone, maybe you can work out a deal with a skilled friend. If you can't trade massages because it irritates your hands, maybe you can substitute something else.

Relaxation Techniques

Lots of people have trouble relaxing, even lying on the physical therapy table. But if you can try to "relax into the pain," you'll speed the healing process.

One of the best relaxation techniques comes from yoga. While lying on the floor, simply tense each part of your body, then let go. This dramatically shows you how much tension you hold even when you're not aware of it. Eventually, you'll learn to let go of tension without having to flex first. You can mentally take stock of your body, find tight spots, and relax them just by using your attention and breath. (For instructions, see the section on deep relaxation, page 117.)

Yoga is great because it is gentle and noncompetitive, and you will be—or should be—told repeatedly not to strain by your teacher. People with severe RSI should avoid certain advanced poses that might strain their forearms, such as the Frog and Handstand. Stick with basic beginner-level poses. Doing yoga can also help calm RSI-induced anxiety.

There are lots of other wonderful relaxation techniques available, including various kinds of meditation. Find one you like and learn how to channel stress safely.

Iontophoresis, Phonophoresis, and Ultrasound

Some methods use sound waves or electrical current to help with pain. In phonophoresis, your rehabilitation therapist will apply a conductive gel and inflammation-reducing medication such as cortisone on your skin, then lightly move an ultrasound device over the painful area. Ultrasound treatments are essentially the same, except no medication is used. The sound waves can be pulsed or constant. Constant waves create heat, which helps reduce pain and increase scar tissue elasticity. If you feel anything other than gentle heat during this treatment, tell your therapist, because bone tissue can be overheated during this process. Iontophoresis is similar to phonophoresis, except electrical stimulation is used to drive medication into the tissue.

Transcutaneous Electrical Nerve Stimulation (TENS)

In transcutaneous electrical nerve stimulation, electrodes carrying low-voltage electricity are positioned along acupuncture points or painful areas on the body. Like ultrasound, this treatment reduces pain, allowing people to move and function in daily life.

NOTE: TENS can worsen reflex sympathetic dysfunction at certain stages. Check with your doctor if this applies to you.

Low-Energy Laser Treatments

Low-energy laser (or cold laser) treatments use light to penetrate the skin to underlying soft tissue, improving circulation by bringing increased blood flow and oxygen to the region. Laser light is thought to help nerve and other cells regenerate and to reduce inflammation.

Upper Body Exerciser (UBE) Machine

Using the UBE is like riding a bicycle with your hands; the machine resembles an exercise bike, except your hands push the pedals instead of your feet. This movement strengthens the entire upper extremity.

PROBLEMS WITH WORK HARDENING

Traditional work-hardening programs, in which the patient was trained to build endurance and strength for work-related tasks, were used when the injury was caused by an accident. Because the work and the work pace both contribute to the problem, work hardening in the context of RSI is inappropriate and could be counterproductive. People can't be hardened to injurious work; the work itself should be changed. "The problem with RSI is that it's not just a medical problem, it's also a management problem," said Jane Bear-Lehman, who teaches occupational therapy at Columbia University. "The medical community can only calm the symptoms." A better, safer approach is a gradual return to work, such as described in Chapter 14.

POSTURE

One of the goals of physical therapy is to teach people the principles of balanced alignment so they are able to incorporate proper posture into all of their daily activities, not just keyboard work. As Michele Semler, a physical therapist at the Miller Institute, noted, "It doesn't do you any good to do a hundred sit-ups in the morning and then walk around with your stomach hanging out all day." You need to exercise good posture consistently.

Good posture plays a crucial role in preventing injury, but bad posture can be extremely difficult to change. Talk to your physical therapist about postural techniques you can practice on your own, such as yoga, the Alexander technique, or other forms of bodywork.

TIP: Put a mirror on your desk so you can monitor your posture while you work. If you glimpse yourself with your chin jutting out, you will be reminded to elongate the back of your neck. You'll also become aware of tension in your jaw or face, which may signal that it is time for a break.

PREVENTIVE EXERCISE

Muscles work in unison, so you must learn to stretch and strengthen corresponding muscle groups to work harmoniously in physical therapy. The classic example of muscle imbalance in computer users is a neck strained forward, rounded shoulders, and a slumped, concave sternum (see Figure 6 on page 27). The overly taut muscles in front pull the shoulders forward, and this causes the muscles in the back to overstretch and weaken. The physical therapist must stretch the tight areas, but the now-relaxed muscle will stay in its new framework only if the corresponding muscles under the shoulder girdle are tightened by strengthening exercises.

To understand how exercise prevents RSI, my patients learn elements of the anatomy and physiology of the arm under the tutelage of the doctors and rehabilitation therapists. We start by explaining the nature of RSI: Thousands of repetitive movements cause microtrauma to muscle tissue, which leads to inflammation. The debris left by inflammation creates scar tissue, which binds down the muscles and strains tendons. Stretching exercises reverse the injury process and promote healing.

Stretching

When I recommend stretching to people, they frequently say that they get up and walk around, or they shake out their hands, mistakenly thinking that these activities ward off RSI. Unfortunately, they do not help. Some folks choose an exercise that exacerbates RSI, such as lifting hand-held weights or doing exercises that strengthen the front chest muscles when they should be stretching them.

Not just any stretching exercise will do. You must learn stretches specific to the affected area. Stretching exercises should be designed for you and supervised by a competent physician or physical therapist.

Overstretching

Overstretching areas that are already too flexible also creates problems, because if one side of the hand, chest, or arm is overstretched, the opposite side is too tight. Patients eventually understand that they should not focus on either stretching or strengthening exclusively; they must focus on both.

POSITIONING

Proper positioning refers to both the correct configuration of the chair and desk and the correct angling of the body to the computer monitor and keyboard. (See Chapters 15 and 16 for advice on this.)

But even perfect ergonomic setups cannot prevent injury unless the people using them are trained to hold their body properly. Every joint has a neutral resting position, at which the muscles and tendons are at their ideal length and operate at optimum efficiency. If someone types in a nonneutral position, the muscles generate less force, fatigue more quickly, and become irritated. Proper positioning should never preclude rest breaks. See Chapter 16 for technique retraining.

PATIENCE

How poor they are that have not patience!
What wound did ever heal but by degrees?

— William Shakespeare, *Othello*

After suffering the relentless abuse of millions of malaligned keystrokes, Nature is slow to forgive the body and allow it to heal. But learning to slow down proves difficult for many patients, who had no idea how long it would take to recover and often feel resentful about this. The path of healing, however, is as subtle as the slow decline into injury, marked by slight improvements, plateaus with no discernable gain, slight relapses, and then more improvements.

The slowness of recovery can be highly frustrating, so when people feel a little better, they try to catch up, push beyond the pain, and wind up having a relapse. "I've had good days and I think, 'Whoopee! I'm on the mend,' and then it comes back," said one woman. The danger here is that reinjury can be worse than the original injury and can happen much more quickly. Psychologically, this sets off a series of unpleasant emotional reactions: People get angry at their jobs, the keyboard, and themselves for ignoring their body's signals and being punished for it. It is also extremely frightening to be so prone to injury. Human nature being what it is, though, a lot of folks have to learn this lesson the hard way before they embrace the habits that will keep them out of trouble.

SIGNS OF HEALING

Signs of healing are as subtle as the arrival of spring. You will be more likely to notice these changes if you keep an RSI log (see page 114). First you might note being pain free at rest; that old soreness just won't seem as bad. Then maybe it won't hurt to push open a door, press the pen through carbon copies, or use an automated teller machine. One patient excitedly announced that she could snap her fingers again for the first time in months. Finally—and this will be late in the game—you might have more endurance. You will become so good at pacing yourself that you won't feel sore at the day's end.

CHAPTER 11

Self-Care: Taking Charge of Your Recovery

My goal is to be as well as I can be. I want to have an active, normal life.

— Woman diagnosed with RSI

Your doctor can only guide your recovery from RSI; the rest is up to you. One of the first things you will learn in rehabilitation therapy is how to care for your hands, arms, shoulders, and neck. This awareness should carry over from computer work into your daily life. You are going to have to train yourself like an athlete in order to use the computer safely. Self-care will make or break your recovery.

Michele Semler, a physical therapist at the Miller Institute, spoke of a star patient who had been seriously injured, but now she is doing well. "When she has pain anywhere, she knows exactly what to do for it," said Semler. The patient knew how to recognize when she was getting tired, stiff, or strained, and she would immediately rest, stretch, or shift position. By paying attention to body cues and attending to them early, she controlled her symptoms. This highly motivated patient learned how to do this for her whole body, not just for the parts affected by RSI. You can learn to do the same thing for yourself.

PAIN MANAGEMENT

If you have RSI, the first thing you need to do is learn to control your pain. When you are in the acute stage of injury, virtually any use of the hand can cause pain. In addition to computer work, handwriting and using a phone or fax machine can trigger symptoms. But most RSI-related pain eventually can be subdued with careful treatment.

Once you pass the acute stage—during which you are in pain almost all the time—you can focus on stretching and strengthening your muscles.

95

Learning from Your Pain

Pain is a great teacher; to master pain, pay attention to it. If something hurts, *stop the offending activity*. Give yourself an ice massage (described below), do some stretches, or just rest. Then go back to work. Repeat this procedure until you learn the subtlest cues and automatically stop *before* the pain begins. Incorporate mini-breaks into your work pattern (see page 184).

Self-Treatment for Pain

You can do a lot to control your pain. My favorite methods for treating pain are simple and benign, relying on the application of ice and heat rather than drugs. You will eventually learn to manage your pain, which not only will make you feel better physically, but will also improve your psychological outlook because it allows you more control over your body.

Ice. Ice is a quick and effective painkiller, and it reduces inflammation and swelling. Because you are in less pain, gentle movement is possible. When you keep moving, you prevent abnormal scar tissue from building, increase blood circulation, and allow proper healing. If you *don't* move, the new tissue is not as flexible as it should be, so it prevents a full range of motion.

Ice should be applied directly to the affected area in short intervals of 40 to 60 seconds, with no more than 10 to 15 icings per day. Apply the ice just long enough to let your skin get numb and red. If you apply ice for too long, the results are the opposite of what you want—you could actually increase inflammation or give yourself an ice burn. "Paint" the ice over painful areas with a massaging motion rather than letting the ice sit in one place. Ice along the painful pathways, concentrating on muscle tissue and avoiding bony spots. Rest your arm on a towel while you do this to catch the drips.

NOTE: Icing is not safe for everyone. If you have circulatory problems, diabetes, Raynaud's syndrome, rheumatoid arthritis, or any other condition that makes you vulnerable to cold, check with your doctor before using ice therapy. Ice can worsen reflex sympathetic dysfunction (see page 58) unless it is applied in the very early acute stages. If you have RSD, do not apply ice unless you have talked to your doctor beforehand.

Don't do stretching exercises or anything strenuous with your hands immediately after icing, because the cold reduces the flexibility of muscles, ligaments, and tendons and they can be injured. Instead, take a 10- to 15-minute break to let your hands and arms warm up again (naturally, don't use artificial means) before you start using them, and go easy in the beginning.

TIP: 1. A handy way to apply ice is to fill a paper cup with water, let it freeze, then rip off the top lip of the cup. Use the cup as an applicator. Put a washcloth or other insulating material around the ice cup to protect your fingers from the cold. After you finish, put the unused portion back in the freezer for next time.

This paper cup method is superior to ice packs because it is cheap and convenient, and a gradual chilling of specific painful areas is preferable to freezing large areas of tissue.

2. Ice sore spots before you retire for the evening.

3. If ice is not available, a cold soda can will work in a pinch. Don't use glass bottles, which could break and cut you.

Heat. Heat can also relieve chronic pain, and it is more appropriate for long-term, rather than acute, injury. Use it for soothing comfort, *not* for treating acute inflammation. Heat can be applied in a heat pack, heating pad, paraffin, warm water, or ultrasound treatments.

Most RSI patients use heat to relax sore neck muscles in a hot bath or shower, or to warm up the hands if they get cold at the keyboard.

Both heat and cold reduce pain in different ways. Here is a rule of thumb regarding the use of heat and cold: *Cold reduces pain; heat assists stretching*. Ask your doctor or rehabilitation therapist if you have questions about when to use heat or cold.

As mentioned above, you should not stretch after icing, but you can safely stretch at room temperature during the day, and a particularly good time for this is after you have had a hot bath or shower.

Hot and Cold Contrast Baths. Hot and cold contrast baths facilitate circulation and are generally advised during the acute phase of injury, sometimes as often as three or four times a day. Contrast baths are believed to improve circulation and are used for people who have swelling.

Instructions

Fill two basins, one with hot (but not scalding) water, one with cold. Soak your hand and forearm for one minute in the cold water. Then soak it for three minutes in the warm bath. Open and close your hands while they are in the warm water only. Repeat this cycle two or three times, ending with the cold bath. Do this on the kitchen counter so you can empty the water basins by spilling them into the sink rather than lifting them.

At work, you can modify this technique using running water from the tap; just be sure the water doesn't scald you. Some people start and end the baths with warm water to facilitate range of motion exercises. Starting and ending with cold water helps reduce swelling.

Stretching

Stretching is one of the best things you can do for yourself now. It brings food (oxygen-rich blood) to muscles, releases tension, reduces pain, promotes healing, and makes you feel good. Stretching also makes you feel young and supple; age need not mean stiffness, though most people make that assumption. You can start stretching—gently—no matter how old you are, and you'll feel great. Just don't overdo it, and be consistent: Stretch every day.

How to Stretch

Most people don't seem to realize that there is a right way and a wrong way to stretch. If you want to know how, observe your pets. Animals do it right instinctively. Even old, arthritic dogs and cats stretch. They don't bounce or stretch halfheartedly; they use slow, steady pressure, and they stop just before they reach the point of pain. After a dog has been curled up for a long time, the first thing it does when it changes position is stretch and shake itself out.

You should do this, too. When you have been sitting at the computer for a long time, do some backward shoulder rolls. Gently look over your shoulder from left to right, and up and down.

Stretch like you mean it, with gradually increasing pressure as you near the limit. If you need help to get the hang of stretching, take a few yoga classes. You will learn how to use your breathing to release tension.

When to Stretch

Stretch frequently during the day. One of my patients timed her stretches to the microwave clock when she heated things up. While the seconds ticked off, she did forearm, neck, and shoulder stretches. This not only made use of otherwise "lost" time; it also reminded her to do her stretches because she used the microwave regularly.

Find moments during the day—including times when you are away from the computer—that work for you. When you take your computer breaks, *get up from the chair* and stretch whatever area feels tight. This could be your back or legs as well as your arms. Pay attention; your body will tell you what needs stretching.

THE IMPORTANCE OF STRENGTHENING EXERCISES

When people are diagnosed with RSI and find out they are injured and their muscles are weak, they almost invariably ask if they should start a strengthening program. There are two reasons for weakness: underuse and overuse. In most cases of RSI, the forearm muscles are overused and the back and shoulder muscles are underused. So don't start lifting weights or doing wrist curls, because those muscles are damaged and need to heal. On the other hand, your rehabilitation therapist will probably start you on strengthening exercises for your back and shoulders right away so they can assist the muscles in your forearms, as they should have been doing all along.

People usually are very enthusiastic about their exercises in the beginning. But the minute they start improving, many people let their home exercise program lapse. They feel like they have licked RSI and they don't have to do their exercises anymore. After they have a couple of flare-ups, they usually mend their ways. Don't make this mistake. Realize how important these exercises are, and do them as though your life depended on it.

Understanding the need for corrective and preventive exercise is one thing; exercising properly is quite another. There is an enormous difference between going through the motions of an exercise and actually working the muscles. Merely imposing rote exercises on people does not work, because they may not understand what they are doing or why and thus may do the exercise improperly. For this reason, you should be carefully trained to notice how your body feels before, during, and after an exercise. Have your rehabilitation therapist explain anything you don't understand so you know the rationale behind your exercise routine.

The learning process varies from person to person: The same set of exercises that takes one person six months to learn could be mastered by someone else in six weeks or six days.

Exercise and postural retraining lead to greater body awareness, so you can respond more quickly to your body's pain signals and learn to use your body more effectively. This is crucial to recovery.

HOME EXERCISES FOR COMPUTER ATHLETES

A good time to do your exercises is first thing in the morning so you get them out of the way and are not tempted to skip them. Be sure to do them every day; if you are not consistent, the exercise will not keep your muscles stretched and toned.

Ask your doctor or rehabilitation therapist for specific instructions before doing any of these exercises. A general rule of thumb is to begin with three

HOLD-UPS

These are so named because you are in the position you see when somebody has been held up in a robbery. The exercise strengthens the upper back and shoulder muscles.

FIGURE 10   Set One.

Lie face down on the floor. Put a pillow under your chest so you can rest your forehead on the floor to avoid neck strain. With your elbows in line with your shoulder, palms face down, elbows bent at a right angle, lift your arms in one unit, keeping everything in the same place as it was on the floor, and slowly pull your shoulder blades together. Pause, then release slowly to the floor and repeat.

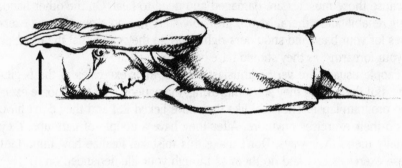

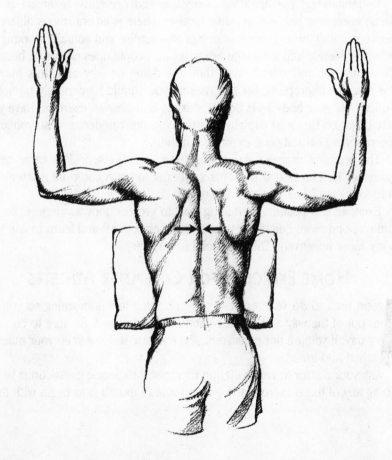

FIGURE 11   Set Two.

Lie face down on the floor as in Set One. With your elbows in line with your shoulder, palms face down, forearms at a right angle to your upper arms, lift your arms in one unit, keeping everything in the same place it was on the floor and pull your shoulder blades together, except this time pull them down toward your tailbone at the same time, with the elbows reaching toward your waist. Pause, then release slowly to the floor and repeat.

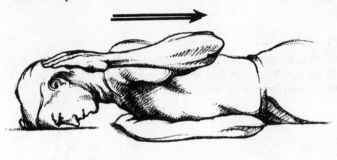

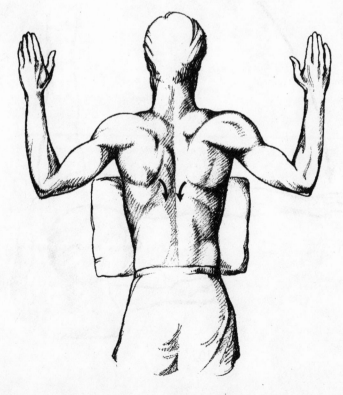

FIGURE 12 The Swimmer.

Lie on the floor with your head facing left so you can breathe. Put your right arm over your head, on the floor, palm down, and your left arm palm down at your side. Now pull both arms up and out. Bring up slowly, pause, and lower slowly. Turn your head, reverse your arms, and repeat to the other side.

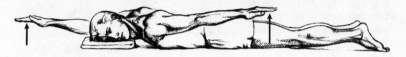

FIGURE 13 Whole Arm Lifts.

Lie on your left side. Bring your right arm in front of your shoulder, palm facing the floor. Slowly raise it from the floor to 90 degrees (but no further, so you don't displace the scapula) and lower it slowly. Repeat to the right.

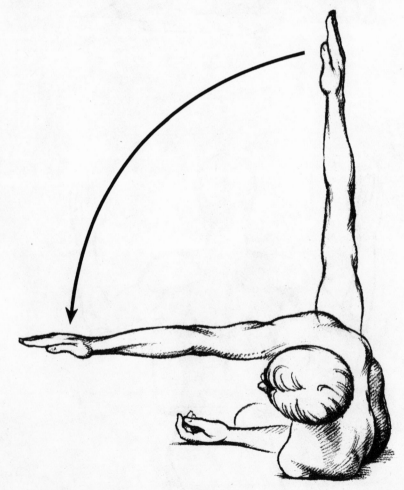

FIGURE 14 Forearm Lifts.

Lie on your left side. With your right elbow touching your waist and arm bent at a right angle, bring your forearm only up to 90 degrees and lower again slowly. Repeat to the right.

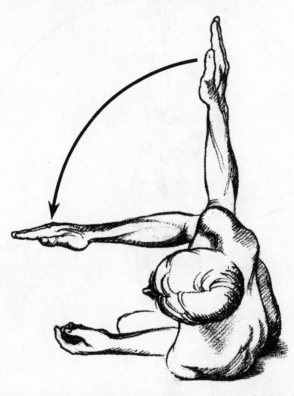

to five repetitions of each exercise, then work up to ten. Add weights *only* if and when your doctor or therapist tells you to do so. With RSI, weights should be wrapped around biceps or forearms, not handheld.

The following routine takes about ten minutes. These are not the only exercises for these muscle groups, so if your physical or occupational therapist has others that you like better, do those. Just be sure these muscle groups get attention.

After your RSI routine, do general loosening or strengthening exercises for your back, legs, abdomen, and other areas. Have your physical or occupational therapist tailor a program for your needs. Your whole body needs to be in good shape for computer work—after all, you might be sitting much of the day, and other areas need attention, too.

NOTE: People ask why they do exercises for their back, shoulder, and neck when their hands hurt. With your new understanding of how the hand works,

FIGURE 15 Arm Circles.
This exercise helps maintain range of motion in your shoulder joint. Lie on your right side. Slowly make ten huge, complete clockwise circles with your arm. Repeat to the right.

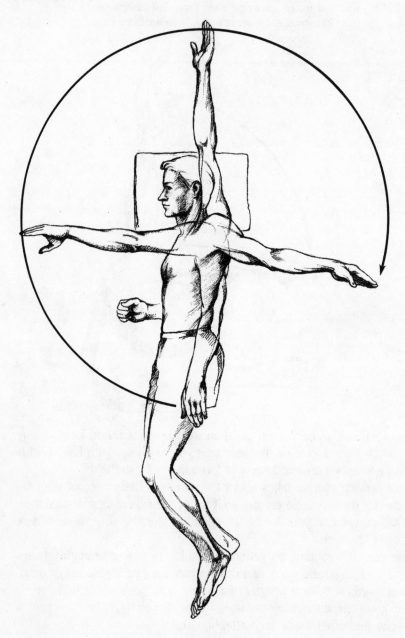

you will understand that the emphasis is on strengthening the more powerful areas to take the strain off your forearms, wrists, and fingers. Stretching is important because a full range of motion gives you better control of your wrists and forearms so the muscles can work efficiently.

OFFICE EXERCISES FOR EYES, NECK, AND PECTORAL AND FOREARM MUSCLES

Here are some exercises for the office. You can do most of them at your desk, but if you prefer more privacy, most restroom stalls are just large enough.

EYE EXERCISES

People tend to neglect their eyes, but the eye muscles become fatigued from staring at the computer screen, too. Here are two exercises that help stretch your eye muscles.

Eyes in a Box (not pictured)

With your eyes straight ahead, look as far to the upper right, lower right, lower left, and upper left corners as you can without straining or turning your head. Reverse directions. Do this three times.

Yoga Clock (not pictured)

The yoga clock is a nice variation.

Looking straight ahead, keeping your head still, imagine a huge clock in front of you. Focus your eyes at high noon, then at one o'clock, two o'clock, and the rest of the hours. When you get to noon again, stop and reverse directions. Do this slowly, without straining.

NECK EXERCISES

Be very careful with any neck exercise, because it is possible to displace a disc in your cervical spine or sprain a neck muscle. Consult your physical therapist or physician before doing these exercises.

Shoulder Circles (not pictured)

Shoulder circles can be done standing or sitting.

Lift your shoulders to your ears, then squeeze them together and down and around to the front again. Make as full a circle as you can.

HEAD TILTS

Sit straight in your chair, with your head in neutral position (Figure 16). Bring your ear to your shoulder without turning your head or lifting the shoulder (Figures 17 and 18). Hold for a count of five. Reverse directions.

FIGURE 16

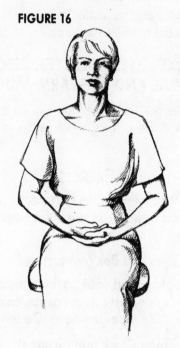

FIGURE 17

FIGURE 18

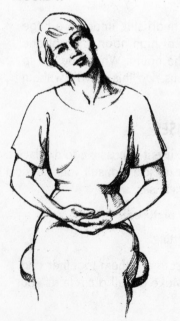

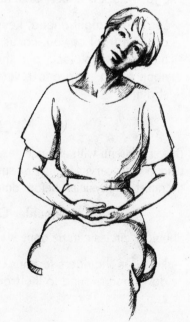

YES'S

Sitting tall, with ears in line with your shoulder, start with your head in neutral (Figure 19), with your focus straight ahead. Then bring your chin toward your chest, stretching the back of your neck (Figure 20). Repeat slowly two times.

FIGURE 19   **FIGURE 20**

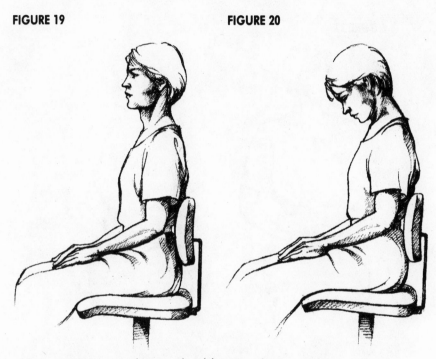

As a variation, circle one shoulder at a time.

Do shoulder circles backward only, because it reminds you to open the front of your chest.

Shoulder Shrugs (not pictured)

Shoulder shrugs can be done standing or sitting.

Lift your shoulders to your ears, hold for a second, and let them drop. Be aware of how relaxed your shoulders feel after you have let them drop.

Shrugs are a quick way to release neck and shoulder tension. They also help increase awareness of tension-holding patterns.

NOTE: Neck rolls, the Yoga Plough, and exercises that require gripping handheld weights or pulleys are not recommended unless you have

NO'S

Start with your head in neutral, as in Figure 16. Without moving your chest or upper back, look all the way to the right (Figure 21). Then look all the way to the left (Figure 22). Repeat slowly two times.

FIGURE 21   **FIGURE 22**

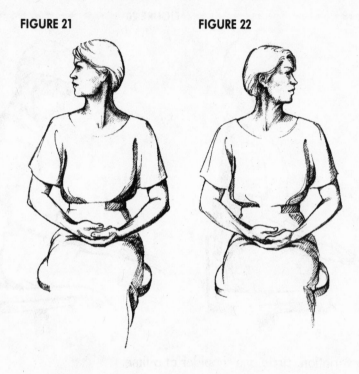

discussed it with your doctor or rehabilitation therapist. These exercises may not harm people in prime condition, but they may strain someone whose muscles either lack tone or are strained and weakened from RSI.

Constructive Fidgeting

There is no one right position in which to sit. Fidgeting, shifting, and even slouching occasionally are normal and good for you. *Any* posture that is rigidly held for a long time is exhausting, even if you are in perfect alignment. Move around while you work: Make tiny adjustments that keep the position dynamic instead of static. Movement will help keep you loose and pain free. Habitual slumping or slouching, however, strains muscles, tendons, and ligaments, so don't do it. Get into the habit of returning to proper alignment after you have shifted away from it.

MOTOWN MOVES

These exercises are designed to stretch your forearms. (The last of these figures looks like a move the Supremes might have made while singing "Stop, in the name of love!"). Be careful not to bend your fingers backward from the tips; instead, support the knuckle joints, as illustrated.

FIGURE 23   Flexed Forearm Stretch.

Hold your arm straight in front of you from the shoulder with the palm facing your body. With your other hand, being careful to keep your fingers over the knuckles of the flexed hand, gently press your hand toward you to a count of ten. Be careful not to raise your shoulder when you do this exercise.

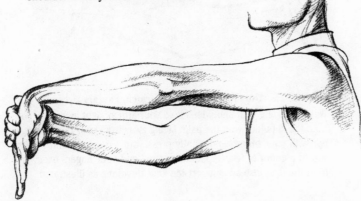

FIGURE 24   Flexed Forearm Stretch with Fist.

Hold your arm straight in front of you from the shoulder, but this time make a fist. With the fingers of your other hand over the knuckles, gently press your fist toward you to a count of ten. Be careful not to raise your shoulder when you do this exercise.

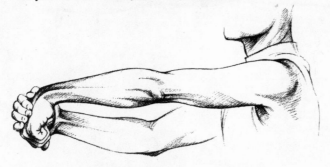

FIGURE 25 Dorsiflexed Forearm Stretch, Fingers Down.

Without raising your shoulders, hold your arm straight in front of you from the shoulder with the palm facing away from your body, fingers down. With your other hand, gently press your hand toward you to a count of ten. Be careful not to bend your fingers backward from the tips; instead, support the knuckle joints, as illustrated.

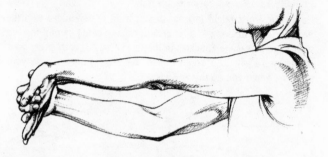

FIGURE 26 Dorsiflexed Forearm Stretch, Fingers Up.

Without raising your shoulders, hold your arm straight in front of you from the shoulder with the palm facing away from your body, fingers up. With your other hand, gently press your extended hand toward you to a count of ten. Be careful not to bend your fingers backward from the tips; instead, support the knuckle joints, as illustrated.

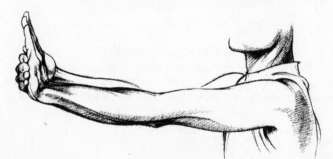

FIGURE 27 Corners.

The hardest part about this exercise will be finding an empty corner. Restroom stalls are readily available and just big enough. Stand about a foot away from the walls. Keep the elbow level with the shoulder and place the entire forearm against the wall. Now lean into it, keeping your spine straight. Hold for ten counts. You'll feel a nice stretch in your pectoral muscles. *Note*: Don't do this with just your hands on the walls, like a push-up. The idea is to stretch your pectoral muscles, so be sure your entire forearm makes contact with the wall, and really lean into it.

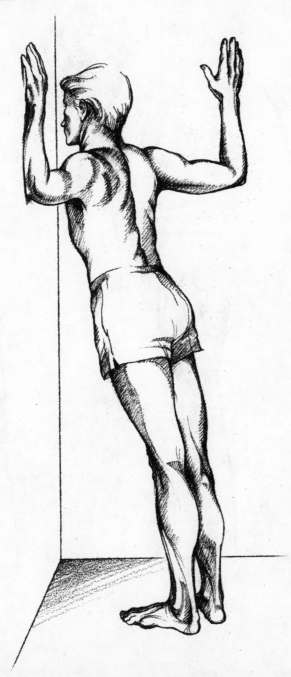

TENDON GLIDES

There are many variations on the tendon glide. Here is one.

FIGURE 28
Starting Position.

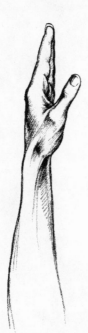

FIGURE 29
Step 1.

Make a fist.

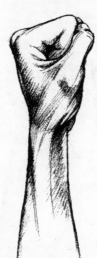

FIGURE 30
Step 2.

Touch your finger-tips to the base of your palm, keeping the thumb straight.

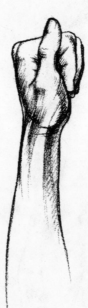

FIGURE 31
Step 3.

Gently make a hook. Don't force your fingers with your other hand if something is painful.

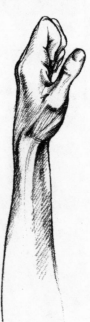

EXERCISE TIPS

- *Pay attention when you do your routine.* Imagine yourself getting stronger, building endurance, and feeling more relaxed with every repetition. Don't do exercises halfheartedly—your mental intent can have a powerful healing effect.

- *Use your exercises to reduce stress.* You will be quiet, unhassled, and calm when you are doing them.

- *If you are self-conscious about doing your exercises at your desk, do them in the restroom.* There is usually exactly enough space to do upper body stretches, and you will be far from prying eyes.

- *Save your favorite exercises for last.* This will motivate you to do the ones you don't like first to get them over with.

- *Form an exercise group at work.* Peer pressure motivates everyone to do their exercises well and to stick to the program.

- *Use music to keep you in rhythm.*

- *Don't shake out your hands.* Violent, whiplike actions do not help and might trigger pain.

- *Think of the total amount of exercise for your whole day.* If you know you are going to be working out your upper body at the gym one day, go easy on your home routine so you don't overdo it.

- *Get a personal trainer.* Some people need a coach to encourage them before they can exercise in groups or on their own, so think about this option if you need extra help or have trouble motivating yourself.

- *Never stretch immediately after icing.* Move gently after application of ice and wait until you've warmed up again before your stretch.

- *Factor in your daily activities.* If you have used your hands vigorously, ease off the strengthening exercises that involve those muscle groups for the day.

OTHER SELF-CARE POINTERS

Don't Let RSI Overwhelm Your Life

Some of my patients are creative about dealing with recovery. One woman limited herself to one RSI-related activity a day, because otherwise she focused on her injury too much. This is a healthy adaptation.

Don't Pressure Yourself

Deadline-oriented jobs can be hazardous to people with RSI, but one smart editor took the pressure off herself by moving everyone else's deadlines up

---

POINTERS ON SELF-CARE

- Pay attention to pain.
- Learn your own symptoms.
- Perform your exercises faithfully.
- Get a massage when you feel like you need one.
- Don't let RSI overwhelm your life.

---

so she wasn't frenzied at production time. If you can even out your work load without overburdening others, do so.

Take Your Time

People who are eager to get well sometimes want to hurry the healing process, but soft tissue injuries such as those associated with RSI heal slowly, and rehabilitation goes slowly, too. It takes weeks and sometimes months of deep tissue massage to remodel scar tissue. If you push yourself—and this can mean anything from typing when you feel pain to straining to open an olive jar—you can relapse into pain. This is understandably very frustrating, but you will soon learn to be careful and respect your limits.

Your recovery will fluctuate like the stock market. You will have good days and bad days during rehabilitation, so don't give up hope if you have a few setbacks. Endurance is the last thing to return, so don't expect to get back to your preinjury level of productivity overnight.

This process takes time, and if you follow the course of rehabilitation faithfully, you will not only improve your chances of getting better, but you will also prevent further injury. There is no quick fix for this injury, but most cases of RSI can be brought under control with a lot of patience and persistence on your part.

OPTIONAL TECHNIQUES

The RSI Log

Keeping a log of your symptoms for a few weeks or months can be a big help. There are two reasons. First, RSI progresses at a creeping rate. Most people don't make a rapid recovery. When you reach a plateau and feel discouraged, you can look back at your diary and see that your symptoms were a lot worse af few months earlier. Second, An RSI log also helps you focus on what you might be doing to aggravate pain, and which self-treatment helps you. Lots of people do not do their exercises regularly, for instance. So in the "possible cause" box, you will see a relationship between your symptoms and not doing your exercises. The same goes for taking breaks, stretching regularly, and not stopping activities that cause pain. Ellen Kolber, an occupational therapist at the Miller Institute, remembers one patient who said that her "hands were killing her" during an occupational therapy session. "I asked her what she had done over the weekend, and she said she had a great time—she went bicycling and rode up a great big hill," Kolber recalled. That patient needed to learn the connection between gripping the handlebars of her bike and her subsequent episode of pain.

Psychologically, keeping a log can give you a sense of control over your condition because you are keeping track of your progress and learning your pain triggers. If it depresses you to look at your symptoms, keeping a running log may not be for you. But if you think it will help, you could set it up in the following way.

Setting Up the Log. The diary is designed to help you better understand yourself and your own symptoms. Use the following as a guide, and feel free to tailor it to your own needs and style. Draw a picture of your arm, neck, and shoulder to show where the pain is. Keep it on your desk so you can note symptoms as they arise. If you do it later, you may forget the subtleties and timing. Keep it until you understand your own symptoms and gain control over the things that trigger them.

1. *Date.* Keeping track of time is difficult, and RSI tends to improve very, very slowly. But if you date your diary, you'll be able to see your progress over time and take encouragement from it, even if it is minor.

2. *Symptoms.* Note your symptoms. Draw a picture of your arm and mark where the pain occurs. Record your pain on a scale of one to ten, ten being the worst pain you have ever felt in your life. This will help you gauge the amount of pain you feel, instead of lumping it all together. Describe the pain, too. Is it aching, burning, shooting? Are you having numbness or tingling? Share this information with your therapist or doctor, because these symptoms may need to be followed up.

3. *Possible Cause.* Can you think of a reason for your pain? Possibilities include forgetting to do your exercises, neglecting to take breaks, working through pain or fatigue, and extra hand-intensive activity during the day. Did you lift heavy groceries earlier in the day? Carry a tray at an awkward angle? Think back. This information

SAMPLE RSI LOG

DATE	Symptoms; Pain 1–10	Possible cause	Action taken	Result	Comments
Oct. 8	Pain in forearm after 1 1/2 hours' work. Pain: 5	Forgot break.	Iced.	Ice helped, but pain came back. Should have taken break on time.	Lots of stress today.
Oct. 10	Pain in forearm; tingling; strain under thumb. Pain: 7	Didn't take break on time.	Stretched.	Felt better, but pain returned upon use of hand.	Worst pain in a long time. Probably holding thumb up to avoid space bar.
Dec. 12	Mild soreness at end of day. Pain: 2	Normal workload.	Remembered breaks and stretches.	Seem to be able to do more with less pain.	No pain on awakening! First time I've noticed this. Can now do dishes again.

will help you avoid stressful activities. Sometimes you will not find a cause, so don't worry if you can't figure out the source of all your pain.

4. *Action Taken.* Noting what you did to reduce the pain helps reinforce good work habits. People know that ice, breaks, and exercise help, but they neglect to do those things.

5. *Results.* Indicate here the effectiveness of the action you took. Was there any change? Was the pain reduced? Did it become worse?

6. *Comments.* Here you make your own notes about things that seem important to you, such as your mood. These will provide insight into how to cope with your symptoms or signs of improvement. Don't focus on just the negative things. The woman who noticed not having pain when she woke up in the morning considered this a great sign of progress; she was right—she had turned a corner in her recovery. Later, she was able to work all day without feeling pain in the evening.

Sharing Your Log. You might want to show your log to your rehabilitation therapist or doctor. They might have important insights or suggestions for you.

Guided Relaxation and Visualization

The purpose of this exercise is to teach you how to relax deeply. This is very good for relieving pain, reducing stress, and healing. Most people don't think they could hold tension in areas of their bodies, such as their eyelids or earlobes, but when you try to relax them, you can actually feel them let go a little.

Progressive relaxation should be done in a quiet environment where you will not be interrupted by noise, ringing phones, or other distractions. Lighting should be soft and indirect; you should not be forced to deal with the glare of overhead lights. You might need a blanket, because you will be deeply relaxed by the time you are through and might feel chilly.

This technique works better if one person talks another person (or group) through the steps, so you can relax completely instead of thinking about the next step. If that is not possible, tape yourself reading the instructions. Many yoga classes have a section devoted to deep relaxation, so you could do that, too.

This section is divided into three parts. As you become accustomed to deep relaxation, guided imagery will be introduced. Finally, desensitization to pain will be attempted to make deep tissue massage easier, if need be.

Progressive Relaxation.

Close your eyes, and let go of all the cares of your daily life. Try to forget about work, or your grocery list, or any other thoughts that enter your mind. Just breathe in and out; every time you exhale, think of letting go of your troubles and tension, and every time you inhale, think of bringing peace and serenity into your body. When you exhale, pain leaves your body, and when you inhale, relaxation and health are restored to all the tissues and nerves and cells of your body.

Let your breathing gradually relax, and as you relax, feel the breath go deeper and deeper, so that you are breathing from your belly rather than your chest. As you relax, let your breathing slow down, and think of the breath as energy that you can direct to any part of your body. This is your own power of relaxation, to use whenever you need it. Just deepen your breath and concentration, and send it to the part of your body that is tense or frightened or in pain, and when you exhale, think of the pain leaving your body and being replaced by good feelings.

If you feel tension anywhere, just direct your breath to go to that area and relax it. If something upsets you or feels too painful, notice it, but move on to another spot. That part may feel better when the rest of your body is relaxed.

Now, starting with your feet, tense and relax different parts of your body. If it is too painful to contract your muscles, just imagine that you are doing it, and let go the same way. Direct your awareness to your feet. Squeeze the toes of your right foot, scrunch your foot into a tight little ball, lift it an inch or so, and let it drop. Then let it find a comfortable resting spot. Now that it is relaxed, let go and forget about it.

Continue with the calf, knee, and thigh, and then do the other leg. Next, start with the fingers, forearms, upper arms, and shoulders on each side, taking care not to strain anything. Then pinch the buttocks together and let them go. Squeeze the shoulder blades together and relax them. Pull in your stomach muscles, and let them go. Relax your intestines. Tighten your pectoral muscles and let them go. Finally, relax your face. Open the jaw wide (gently), and then relax it. Purse your lips. Wrinkle your nose. Squeeze your eyelids shut. Then relax, and relax anything else you've missed.

Now enjoy the sensation of being perfectly at peace for a while. In a few moments, you can gently wake up your body, and it will probably feel refreshed, rested, and less painful. Whenever you need to, you can come back to deep relaxation to restore yourself to harmony.

When you have practiced this technique for a while, you can reach a deeply relaxed state in less time.

Visualization.   Go through deep relaxation, as described above.

Now that your body is fully relaxed, you can forget about it and just let it sink into the floor, and allow the forces of gravity support it. Though your body is fully relaxed, your mind is very alert and active.

Imagine that golden light is entering your body, and that the light will heal all the parts that hurt. The warm light enters from the top of your head, and it gently dissolves pain as it goes along. Let the light travel down your neck and into your (right or left) arm. Any time you feel any pain, pause there for a minute, and gently breathe into that spot. Notice the pain change, and the relaxation that can result.

Slowly direct your awareness down your arm, and let the healing energy warmly dissolve pain. Now visualize your shoulder joint, and imagine the joint moving freely, without pain. Imagine that your biceps and triceps muscles are toned and responsive and strong. Imagine that your forearm muscles are long and smooth and elastic. All of your muscles are getting stronger, and as they get stronger, they move freely and easily.

Send your attention to your wrists, and imagine that they are protected by the strength and elasticity of your forearm. All of your muscles, from your back to your shoulder blades, your biceps and triceps and forearm muscles will evenly distribute the load, allowing your fingers to move easily through work. Your strong muscles support your fine movements, and you protect yourself from pain, as though you had an invisible golden shield on your arm. This shield is formed by your own strong, toned, and stretched muscles, and it allows you to move freely and easily without pain.

Now go even deeper into your body, and imagine the cells of your bones and tendons and muscles healing. All the painful cells are breaking down and being replaced by healthy ones. Your blood is getting fresh oxygen from your breath and carrying away all the toxic materials from the old cells. With each breath, you are creating healthy new cells; with each exhalation, damaged cells are floating away.

This is a good thing to do at night, before you go to sleep.

Desensitization for People Who Have Pain during Massage. After you are comfortable with guided relaxation and visualization, try this. The intent is to help you relax during deep tissue massage. Tell your rehabilitation therapist if anything hurts or doesn't feel right. It is okay if something "hurts good," though. Show your massage therapist this exercise so you can work on it together.

Start very slowly. You might want to ask your massage therapist not to touch you for a while, but rather talk you through the process in imagination until you feel ready for the real massage. Imagine that it is painless and makes you feel better. Remember, you are in control, and if something is too painful, you can ask your therapist to use lighter pressure, move from that area, or stop entirely.

Start with deep relaxation technique. When you are relaxed, start this visualization.

Imagine that you are receiving a light massage. Every time your therapist massages a muscle, it will feel like pain leaves your body and is replaced by a feeling of warmth and well-being. You and your therapist are both doing the massage, in a sense: While the therapist uses his or her hands to improve range of motion and remodel scar tissue, you are helping by relaxing and directing your breath to the area being worked on, releasing the tension that is being held in that area.

You can try this on your own if you are too shy to tell your rehabilitation therapist that you are uncomfortable having massage. If you are comfortable with your therapist, you can work out your own script.

Some rehabilitation therapists have a good knack for calming people down: They will talk to you during the massage to help distract you from unpleasant feelings.

Relaxation Works Better with Practice. Most people feel great after deep relaxation but don't do it consistently even though it helps them. Pleasant as it is, it takes practice, so make time for it if you want greater benefits.

CHAPTER 12

Activities of Daily Living

I finally convinced my landlord to allow me to have a garage door opener in-stalled (at my expense)....I think the key persuasion factor was letting him know the garage door had blown shut (literally on me and/or my car) on more than one occasion.

— Robin Coutellier, *RSI Network*

You'll hear your doctor and rehabilitation therapist use the phrase "activities of daily living" (or ADLs) frequently; the phrase refers to simple things such as brushing your teeth and hair, putting in contact lenses, cutting vegetables, opening doors, and turning faucets. The ADLs are one of the best ways to judge the severity of an injury, and information about how you perform them is a valuable part of your diagnosis, both for showing the extent of injury and showing how much you have improved from therapy and exercise.

Having to restrict your ADLs is the reason being disabled by RSI is so difficult: No one wants to feel helpless or be forced to have to rely on other people for simple tasks such as buttoning jeans or cutting food.

TRICKS FOR BETTER LIVING

If you have RSI, there are a number of ways you can make life easier. A few ideas are included here to get you started, but you will certainly devise your own favorites. You will be inspired by various sources: your occupational therapist, other people you know who have RSI, and reading about it.

AT HOME

Negotiate Chores

Housework has probably caused more domestic arguments than politics, and some people with RSI seethe when nobody helps with the work they used to do alone. You want a clean house when the rest of your life is in shambles. If your family is willing to pitch in and take over things you used to do, that's wonderful. If not, you have a problem, because you shouldn't—

or can't—do a lot with your hands. One woman said, "I was so furious at my kids for not helping me. I thought, I'll just do it myself." But she aggravated her injury this way, which made her situation worse.

"Getting the kids to do something starts with the spouse," said Dr. Robert Rosenthal, a San Francisco Bay area psychiatrist. "The kids won't help if they see the husband not lifting a finger to help. Single moms need to sit down and have a serious talk with their kids." Obviously, household chores should be assigned according to the age of the child. Children should not be forced into the role of caretakers and caregivers. Enlist the aid of your physician or psychotherapist to help get kids and spouse to cooperate.

One gambit for negotiating chores is to ask for volunteers: If someone loves to iron, put that person in charge of the laundry, and let him off the hook for chores he dislikes. Use paper plates, or have housemates do their own dishes. Choose one room that you spend a lot of time in and keep *that* room in shape; let the rest go for a while.

But try not to push yourself too hard. If your kids are uncooperative, don't take the entire burden upon yourself. You may have to lower your standards about housework until you get better.

Hire Household Help

If you have the money, it is obviously better to hire someone to help you with chores that bother your hands, such as mopping, vacuuming, or doing laundry, than doing it yourself.

See about Home Care

If you don't have the means to hire household help, you may qualify for home care through your local social service department. (See the Resources section on page 208.)

Don't Do It All in One Day

Rather than going off on a cleaning frenzy, spread the heavy work out over the week; if Monday is laundry day, don't scrub the walls and do all the vacuuming, too. Spread your chores out over the day as well.

Do Chores More Often

Think about ways you can do things more often that will reduce the amount of physical force you will need to use. For example, mop the floor frequently so you don't need to scrub it. Soaking pots and pans so they don't need scouring is also useful. Grocery shopping and laundry are hard on the hands, so do these chores more frequently to lighten the burden.

Electrify

Use electric staplers, knives, scissors, can openers, and erasers.

How to Open a Door

Most people with RSI learn this without needing to be told: Don't push the door open with your hands; instead, lean into it with your forearm and your body weight. For a heavy door with a lock, hold it open with a foot, rather than a hand, and *then* push it open with your hip and thigh or shoulder.

How to Read a Book

Book lovers are frequently dismayed when they realize they can't open books or hold them up anymore. When you get a new book, if it offends you to crack the spine so the pages stay open, try this method: Hold open the first page, and then crease the pages open at the center. Or use a clip or leather thongs with weights on either end to hold both pages open. Public libraries also carry books on tape, so you can listen rather than read. (See page 209 for more taped books.)

Reading in bed is not recommended, because it usually requires you to crane your neck; reading in a good chair will allow you to maintain better positioning. However, if one of your life's greatest pleasures is reading in bed, prop the book on a pillow or bookstand, and balance your poor posture with exercise. You might also like using a bookstand or pillow while reading at a table so you can get the right angle without using your hands.

Reading in bed is a perfect example of the kind of trade-off to which people with RSI need to become accustomed. If you know you are straining your neck to do something that gives you pleasure, you need to make a compromise: Limit the amount of time you read in bed, and be sure to balance this less-than-desirable posture with exercise and stretching. "Everybody's got a list of things they just grit their teeth and do," said Jane Bear-Lehman, who is an assistant professor of clinical occupation therapy at Columbia University. Decide for yourself what your priorities are and give up things that are less important.

Your Pillow

Your pillow can be more important than you might think, because sleeping in the wrong position can affect your alignment. If you sleep on your stomach (which is not advisable, but it is the only way some people can fall asleep), you shouldn't use one because it puts your neck out of alignment. If you sleep on your side, you might need two in order to keep your neck bones in line.

Play with your pillows: Does your arm feel more comfortable when you slip a pillow under your arm? If you like the idea of a cervical pillow (which supports your neck but has a well for your head), try making your own: Roll up a towel and place it lengthwise at the bottom of the pillowcase.

Other Sleep Tricks

Try to train yourself to sleep with your elbow straight to avoid numbness and tingling that can come when the elbow is bent. Talk to your doctor or occupational therapist if you think you need a splint to prevent you from flexing your wrist at night. Soft splints are available.

IN THE KITCHEN

Opening Things

Use pliers, rubber pads, or commercial jar openers to help you open jars. (A rubber glove works in a pinch for added traction.) Break the seal with a can opener rather than forcing the lid open with your hands. Use pliers to pull off tabs from juice or soda cans and loosen tight caps. Run hot water over metal caps to loosen them.

To open a jar with one hand, put the bottom in a drawer and hold it shut with your hip to keep the base of the jar stationary while you undo the lid.

Knives

Keep knives sharp for easier cutting. Look for ergonomically designed knives; make sure they are high quality and well balanced. Two-handled knives balance the work between your hands. Consider an electric knife if you have trouble carving meat.

Don't use kitchen knives to open jars, plastic bags, or packages. Use scissors for plastic bags; it's safer.

Scissors

Buy scissors with spring-loaded or loop handles for easier cutting. Open plastic bags, cereal pouches, and foil packages with scissors instead of knives.

Utensils

Look for measuring spoons with long handles that are easy to grasp, measuring cups with handles you can slide your hand under to hold securely, graters with suction feet that will stay put while you use them, battery-operated whisks, and mixing bowls with nonskid bases.

Use two-handled casserole dishes and vegetable steamers—they are safer to lift than those without handles. Use small containers—they are easier to lift and clean. Get easy-to-hold handles for the milk carton. Use pumps for the catsup so you don't have to shake the bottle. Make sure handles on pots are long, easy to hold, and sturdy.

Consider buying a food processor to make food preparation easier—but be sure you can assemble and disassemble it *before* you buy it!

See the Resource section on page 209 for catalogs that sell ergonomic kitchen aids.

Kitchen Techniques

Use *both* hands for tasks such as lifting heavy or hot pots, opening milk cartons, and carrying trays. Position mixing bowls in the corner of the sink when you use the hand mixer to avoid holding the bowl.

To avoid having to squeeze the handle of a sifter, put flour in a strainer and rub it through with a spoon. Crank-handle and battery-operated sifters are also available.

Transfer heavy things such as catfood, milk, and detergent from big containers to little ones. If you don't have an automatic ice cube maker, fill the tray only half full with water for easier removal of ice cubes.

Adapting Your Kitchen

If you remodel your kitchen, position the range and oven at the same height as the counter so you can slide, rather than lift, heavy pots. Make sure the counter is the proper height. When you bend over your work, it stresses the back, neck, and shoulders.

Use open shelving, or be sure that the cabinet door handles are easy to use. The same goes for faucets: Look for ease of use. There is nothing more frustrating than glitzy hardware that is difficult to operate. Adaptive handles are available through catalogs (see the Resources section, page 209).

Install your oven at counter height to avoid back and arm strain. Use shallow shelves to avoid having to lift one object to get another. Get a double sink. Lifting a heavy dishpan is hard work. Store heavy things, such as flour jars, where you can slide, rather than lift, them.

YOUR SEX LIFE

People rarely speak of sexual problems that result from RSI, but not being able to use your hands, or have someone touch them, without pain can hinder lovemaking. RSI can be particularly problematic for anyone who receives affection only during intercourse. Other people can become extremely depressed and give up sex altogether because of complex emotional reactions to injury. Maybe they feel that the possibility of love and romance is gone. According to Clark Taylor, a sexologist on the staff of the Institute for Advanced Study of Human Sexuality, "The feelings per se need to be gone through. They are not your sex life—they are your feelings."

Rather than dealing with those issues right away, you might want therapy to get at the underlying feelings; in any case, try not to despair. Having RSI does not have to end your sex life. In fact, if you play your cards right, it could be better than you ever imagined. If you are embarrassed to ask your doctor for sexual advice, talk to your psychotherapist, see a sex therapist, or do some reading—there are lots of good books available on this topic.

You Are Not Alone

You aren't the only person whose sex life has suffered from an injury or illness. As Dr. Taylor has pointed out, women who have had mastectomies need to substitute other parts of their bodies for the joy they used to receive from their breasts. "Quadriplegics can lose sensation in their genitals, so they learn to become orgasmic in other parts of their bodies, such as the top of their head," he added. So don't feel like you have to give up your sex life just because you have RSI—you just need to find new techniques.

Communicate and Explore Your Options

Good communication is crucial when it comes to sexual matters. Are you lying there in pain for your partner's pleasure, or can you say it hurts? Can you let your partner know that you still enjoy being cuddled even if it is too painful to do more than that at the moment? Be specific; sensitive lovers do not want to cause pain.

Use RSI as an opportunity to explore different things you've never needed to try before. You will probably find richer avenues of sensuality than you thought possible.

Making Love without Hands

Making love without hands is possible. Start by looking at what you *can* use. Maybe your hands hurt, but what other parts of your body can you use? Our entire body is highly sensitive to touch; most people miss this fact because they are so focused on their genitals.

Nonsexual Touch

There are nonsexual ways to help ease tensions that shouldn't be ignored. Treat yourself to a massage. This is especially beneficial to those who are not assertive about their sexual needs: It is a chance to receive physical pleasure instead of feeling compelled to please a partner. If it hurts to have your hands massaged, have your therapist work on your feet or other body parts.

Pamper yourself. Is there anything you can do within the boundaries of your pain to experience pleasure? Do warm, perfumed baths make you feel good? What about getting a facial, sauna, or a pedicure? Lots of people find that their arms feel better after they have had an aerobic workout; one woman said the only time her arms didn't hurt was during sex. Try to find something that makes you feel good and takes your mind off RSI.

IN THE CAR

When you drive, your car becomes your workstation, and it can exacerbate RSI. Look at ways you can improve ergonomics: Will a lumbar curve cushion (or a rolled-up towel) reduce back or neck pain? Is your seat pulled close enough to the brake and gas pedal to avoid a long reach?

Here are some other driving tips:

- *Don't lean on your armrest while you drive.* It can irritate the ulnar nerve.

- *Don't hold the steering wheel too tightly.* Padded steering wheel covers are easier to hold.

- *When you buy a car, judge the ergonomics.* Is the steering wheel wide enough? A shoulder-width apart is good. Small steering wheels tend to cause people to pull their shoulders forward. Are the door and window handles easy to open? Is the seat well designed and easy to adjust?

- *Don't drive for more than 30 to 45 minutes without getting out of the car and stretching.* You will feel much better when you arrive at your destination if you do this. Trade off with another driver on long journeys.

PERSONAL CARE

Fingernails

Keep your fingernails short. Long nails make it difficult to use your hands effectively. Use a suction-cup nail brush if you have trouble holding things.

Hair

Some people choose a short haircut that requires little brushing or styling. Mount your blow-dryer so you don't have to hold it to dry or style your hair.

THE MEDICINE CABINET

Childproof caps can be nearly impossible to open for people with RSI. If you don't have small children, talk to your pharmacist about avoiding them. Use a tool to undo lids rather than straining your fingers, and keep a spare tool in the medicine cabinet.

YOUR BUYING HABITS

Buy Smaller Sizes

The large economy size of detergent is not a bargain unless you can get someone else to carry it home and transfer it to a smaller container for pouring. Shop more frequently rather than carry heavy loads home.

Don't Accept Inferior Design

Don't be a passive consumer of dreadful industrial design. We can all develop our intuitive grasp of good design, and ironically, people with RSI are probably the best judges of all, because poor design will trigger their symptoms. Use your special knowledge of what strains your hands to guide your purchases.

Start noticing the handles and buttons on tools. A spray dispenser with a handle on the side that can be grasped with several fingers will be easier to use than one with a button on top, which requires downward pressure to operate.

Look for ergonomic tools. There are special designs for knives, carpentry tools, and scissors. Check them out. (See the Resources section, page 209.)

Adapt Your Tools

Use your ingenuity to adapt existing tools to fit your hands better. Ask your occupational therapist for advice about design and tool modifications.

AT THE OFFICE

Telephone Headsets

If you work while you are on the phone, get a headset. You risk serious injury by holding the phone with your shoulder. Speaker phones are great, too, but only for the speaker. Unfortunately, for the person on the receiving end of the conversation it sounds like you're shouting in a tunnel, which is why using them is considered bad telephone etiquette. Speaker phones are not great for conversations you wish to be private, either.

Headsets allow both you and your listener to have a comfortable conversation. Use them both at home and at the office if you use your hands while you talk.

Automatic Dial and Redial

Pressing a touch-tone phone is painful if you have RSI. Program frequently dialed numbers and take advantage of automatic redial to save your hands.

Fat Pens

Write with a fat pen that you don't have to grip. You can transform a skinny one with a foam hair curler, or get a pen expander at the stationer's. Some people prefer felt-tipped pens because they don't require a lot of downward pressure; others dislike the drag of the fibers. Choose a pen that is comfortable for you: Avoid pens you must grip or press to use. Make photocopies if it hurts to press through carbons.

Gloves

Giving advice about gloves is tricky. Gloves take away normal sensation, which you need to protect your hands from harm, but gloves may protect your hands in some circumstances. If you wear gloves, make sure they fit properly and have rubberized or leather treads to supply traction at the palm. Ill-fitting gloves can cause pressure on the nerves between the fingers. If your gloves don't give you enough traction to get a good hold on things, you may grip too hard.

Fingerless wool gloves may be helpful if your hands get cold; just make sure they don't choke your fingers. "Support" style gloves work rather like splints, so don't work while wearing them.

SAFE CARRYING TECHNIQUES

You don't realize how much carrying you do until you get RSI. If you are severely injured, carry as little as possible, because it strains your hands. Here are a few suggestions.

Use Wheels

Carrying things can challenge people with RSI. Lugging heavy grocery bags with handles can strain your hands, but so can cradling them in your arms. Use wheeled carts to transport heavy loads, such as your briefcase, laundry, or your suitcase, if you are traveling. Carrying something heavy during a stressful situation such as trying to catch a plane could lead to a relapse.

Get Rid of Your Shoulder Bag

Use belt bags instead of carrying a purse or wearing a shoulder bag. Heavy shoulder bags strain your neck muscles, because you tense them to keep the strap from slipping off; they also cause your posture to be unbalanced. If you must wear a shoulder bag, keep it light; shift it from side to side periodically or cross the strap over your chest to distribute the load more equally.

Backpacks can be good for some people, depending on their injury and pain level. Talk to your occupational therapist before you start using one. Look for light weight; wide, padded shoulder straps; and a belt support to distribute weight evenly.

SPORTS AND RECREATION

Your rehabilitation therapist should ask you about your hobbies and recreational activities to get an idea of how else you might use (or unwittingly abuse) your hands during the day. Occupational therapists are trained to help you adapt your environment to be less stressful, so be sure to ask lots of questions about improving your ergonomics.

Adapt Your Activities to Accommodate Your Injury

Exercise. Exercise is an important component of good health. If you don't have an exercise program, ask your physical or occupational therapist about starting one. You will need exercise more than ever if you are injured—to help keep your cardiovascular system strong, and as a stress reducer. Don't think you have to stop exercising just because you're injured. One woman was most distressed at thinking she would have to discontinue using her cross-country ski machine, which helped her stay in shape. I suggested she wear the harness on her biceps rather than holding them with her hands so she could keep exercising. Another woman wore splints while she swam to ensure that she wouldn't ulnar deviate. Talk to your occupational therapist about safe adaptations to your current regimen.

Bicycling. If you enjoy cycling, look at the handlebars on your bike. If they are low and put your hands in dorsiflexion, you will have to make adjustments. Ergonomic handlebars exist. You can also buy tubing to make handlebars bigger and more comfortable. This is useful for other sports equipment as well. Fingerless cyclists' gloves can help you keep your grip.

At the Gym. Be careful which machines you use: If they require hand-intensive effort, don't use them. Don't use hand-held weights unless you

---

DOS AND DON'TS

- Do use your big joints and muscles to do the work, not the little ones.
- Do use tools for force, not your hands. Keep an extra set of pliers or a screwdriver in the kitchen and medicine cabinet so you will be inclined to use a tool to open things rather than forcing them with your hands.
- Do buy clothes with elastic waistbands, or shoes with Velcro straps or other streamlined features. They are easier to put on than those with tricky zippers, buttons, snaps, or hooks.
- Don't be foolish with your hands. You wouldn't be careless with your heirloom crystal or your camera, so don't use any less caution with your hands.
- Don't pound the stapler.
- Don't pry off the cap with your hands.
- Don't do heavy lifting.

---

have been advised to do so by your physician or a competent rehabilitation therapist.

Watch Which Exercises You Do

Tell your rehabilitation therapist what kinds of exercises you do, because they may be counterproductive at this point. If you tend to slump your shoulders, play down the exercises that strengthen the pectoral muscles and concentrate on exercises that tighten the scapula. You may need to alter your program to get your muscles back in balance.

Be Aware of Your Total Daily Exercise

If you do a heavy gym workout, you may have to cut down your daily RSI exercise routine that day. Overdoing exercises or stretches can stress your muscles—the thing that probably gave you RSI in the first place. Factor in your total exercise for the day, and don't do too much.

HELP FOR THE PERMANENTLY/PARTIALLY DISABLED

If you have been permanently or partially disabled by RSI, you may qualify for help from community, state, or federal agencies. This could include counseling, assistive devices, vocational training, home care, and even home modification. (See the Resources section, page 208.)

You may need to meet eligibility requirements, however, and if you are well-off financially, you may have to pay for some of the services. One of the things an agency might do, for instance, is retrofit a kitchen, replacing hardware to allow a person self-sufficiency at home. It may also provide education or vocational training, and perhaps even a voice-activated computer. It is definitely worth a call if you think you need that kind of help. However, bear in mind that the efficiency of government bureaucracies varies from state to state and community to community. RSI may not be recognized as a disability; you may have to be persistent to get help.

Check the Resource Section at the back of this book for more information.

CHAPTER 13

Your Emotions

All pain is in your head. You feel it in your brain.

— Robert Rosenthal, psychiatrist

THE EMOTIONAL IMPACT OF RSI

Any serious illness can unleash a tempest of emotional reactions, and RSI is no exception. Psychological reactions can result from the injury: Because they have been injured, people feel angry; because they can no longer use their hands, they feel frustrated and impotent. Psychological problems that existed before the onset of RSI can become worse.

The hand has enormous significance in life and profound psychological implications. Phrases such as "My hands are tied," "I can't handle it," and "Get a grip!" aptly describe feelings of powerlessness or loss of control that result from not being able to use your hands.

The inability to use one's hands has even more sinister implications: "In Elizabethan times, people were punished by being ridiculed in public squares held by the wrists in stockades," noted Robert Markison. "Now, we restrain criminals with handcuffs." Perhaps the most poignant image of all is the final reflex of the man facing the firing squad, raising his hand in a futile attempt to stop the bullets.

What makes RSI particularly difficult to deal with is that your emotional state can affect symptoms. It helps to stay upbeat.

Keeping your emotions steady when your finances, job, and family life have been shattered can be nearly impossible to do alone. If you have close, supportive friends or a spouse who will listen to you, you are blessed. But if you don't have someone whose shoulder you can cry on—or if your friends and family are not coming through for you—don't feel you have to bear this burden by yourself. Enlist the aid of a good psychiatrist or psychologist, or join a support group. "I feel like all I talk about is my injury," one woman ruefully admitted. If you don't want to feel like a whiner with friends, take advantage of sympathetic listeners who *want* to hear all about it.

Seeking Emotional Support Is Not a Sign of Weakness

Even in this supposedly enlightened day and age, asking for help with handling your emotions is often seen as a sign of weakness. People view seeking emotional help as a sign that they are "crazy" or weak. Nothing could be further from the truth. Seeking psychological counseling is a sign of great courage, and those who do often go far in life, because they are able to put self-defeating behavior behind them instead of repeating old patterns. "Part of the problem is that doctors only refer people to psychiatrists when they feel there is nothing else they can do," observed Robert Rosenthal, a West Coast psychiatrist who specializes in people with chronic pain caused by hand injuries. "This is not about being crazy. Any illness has emotional consequences, and the better you cope with the emotions, the better you'll cope with the illness itself."

To compound the problem, people sense—often correctly—that their doctors or rehabilitation therapists don't want to hear about their problems. I have heard some health professionals impatiently refer to patients who do talk about their problems as "mental cases." Perhaps this intolerance arises from their own inability to deal with chronic pain. On the other hand, if concerned health providers advise a troubled person to see a psychologist in a sincere effort to help, and that suggestion is ignored, the health providers' sense of frustration seems justified.

THE FIVE STAGES OF DEALING WITH RSI

Human emotion is far too complex to generalize about here, and it would be simple-minded to paint a portrait of the "RSI personality." However, there are certain emotional stages that many people seem to go through when they develop RSI. Of course, not everybody goes through all of them.

The First Stage: Denial

The first stage is usually denial, which means that instead of paying attention to pain or other symptoms, people shrug them off. This does not refer to people who went to the doctor and were told nothing was wrong, or people who had no idea that RSI existed and would have been willing to deal with it had they known. Awareness about RSI is not common, so people cannot be blamed for not knowing what to do.

Denial in this sense refers to people who deny they have a problem until their condition becomes severe. It is normal to shrug off the fleeting aches and pains of daily life, but some people shatter every glass in the house before they finally admit that they can no longer hold on to things.

In the beginning, most people are not even aware that they are denying that a problem exists. You will see them massaging their wrists or shaking out their hands because their fingers have fallen asleep, and if you say, "Gee, maybe you should see a doctor," they will say, "No, I don't have RSI. This happens all the time, but it goes away." Or "I've been typing this way for years, and nothing has ever happened."

Fear also pays a big role in the denial stage. Many people with severe symptons of RSI put off seeing a doctor because they are afraid they will lose their jobs. This view is realistic but shortsighted: A job can be replaced, but if you lose your hands, you may be *permanently* unemployable and permanently disabled.

A false sense of security is another form of denial. One reporter who had RSI said that she had gone to a doctor right away and put some corn pads on her keyboard to soften the touch. When I described the techniques we recommend to prevent injury, such as taking breaks and pacing, she said, "Oh, that's impossible. My editor's always breathing down my neck. We don't have time for breaks. Can't do it. No time."

She seemed to think that because she had gone to the doctor and got a diagnosis, she was automatically protected from further injury. But corn pads will not help if you never take breaks. She did not seem to see her own crucial role in preventing her condition from getting worse. If her editor is unreasonable and refuses to allow her to take breaks, she has a real problem: She might feel justifiably terrified of losing her job. On the other hand, she might be driving herself harder than necessary because of internal pressures. Maybe her editor wouldn't mind if she took breaks. But here we need the cooperation of labor and management, and that can be tricky. Sometimes management adopts the attitude that your doctor will take care of it, but your doctor cannot take care of that part of RSI because the doctor isn't the one doing your job: He can't pace himself or do your exercises for you. Denial is dangerous, because the longer you let your symptoms go, the greater the risk of permanent injury.

The Second Stage: Panic

Eventually, most people break through denial, go to a doctor, and are diagnosed. Then comes the second stage: panic. People imagine the worst: losing their jobs, losing their houses, and permanently losing use of their hands.

Panic can be positive if it motivates people to "do something" to get better, but most people have no idea how long it takes soft tissue injury to heal, and the last thing they want to hear is advice on patience, pacing, and exercise, which are the best things they can do for themselves.

The Third Stage: Anger

I think of the computer as the enemy right now.

— Woman with RSI

Once people realize that they have injured themselves—and that they aren't getting better quickly—the next emotion they face is rage. They are angry at their boss for being too demanding, their company, their doctor, their coworkers, and the keyboard.

When you are angry, your pain can feel worse, and you are likely to injure yourself further—by not looking where you're going and stubbing your toe, for instance. Treat anger as a warning signal that you need to take action. First, recognize that you are angry. Accept the anger. Then think about what you can do about the situation that provoked it. For instance, if your doctor refused to listen to you during an examination and walked away after two minutes, you could bring it up with him, or you could see another doctor.

There are helpful and destructive responses. Just raging is destructive. If you are angry about something specific, take action. If it is just general rage, acknowledge it and talk to someone. RSI groups are good for this sort of thing. It is appropriate to be angry at this stage, and it will pass. Don't take your anger out on yourself by forgetting to pace yourself or pounding the keyboard—you will only hurt yourself.

The Fourth Stage: Depression

Depression and anger are closely related, and many people with RSI—particularly those with very serious injuries—fall into deep despair. This depression is often related to the loss of being able to do things for yourself. To cope with depression, combat a sense of helplessness by focusing on what you *can* do. Try to make it something active rather than passive.

If you are so depressed that you can't get out of bed in the morning, or if you have thoughts that life may not be worth living, you may need medication to give you a boost until you can get some perspective. This does not imply that you will be on drugs for life: they are meant to be used to get you over the hump. After that, you go off the medication.

The Fifth Stage: Mastering RSI

Now we come to the turning point. This is where things get really interesting, because so much depends on individual reactions. After going through all these emotions, some people get stuck in vicious depressions. They focus on what they can't do, or how angry they are at Workers' Comp. RSI fills their entire mental horizon.

Other people get depressed for a while, but then they seem to suspend their anger, accept the fact that they have RSI, and start figuring out how to deal with it. It is similar to watching ballet dancers working on their technique. They will be totally rapt, slowly doing a certain step or turn over and over, analyzing it move by move, and trying to make it perfect.

People with RSI do the same thing. They start experimenting with how they sit. They stop and consider what happened when something hurts, and learn their own triggers. The RSI log is extremely useful here.

At this stage, people develop positive coping mechanisms. One woman turned off the television after the first two months she was out on disability. She didn't want to start thinking of herself as disabled and that all she could do was watch television.

This is when people start mastering RSI. If they can get a toehold, and maybe have a good day, they take courage and the tide turns in recovery.

RSI DOESN'T HAPPEN IN A VACUUM

Preexisting Emotional Problems

RSI is also complicated because it doesn't occur in a vacuum. If you have preexisting emotional problems, and were depressed, angry, or upset about something *before* you were injured, dealing with RSI may be tougher for you than someone for whom things were going smoothly.

Sense Memory

The body is capable of storing the memory of trauma for years. Sometimes this sense memory actually molds the shape of the body, as in the case of a man whose parents struck him in the face as a child and now literally walks with a "chip on his shoulder"—with one or both shoulders held defensively high. This phenomenon can make recovery from RSI doubly difficult for some people, especially those with prior unresolved emotional problems from childhood. If someone has been physically or sexually abused, it may be difficult to receive deep tissue massage in physical therapy, because of a deep fear of being touched.

"Injury memory remains in the tissues well after the damage is done," noted Robert Markison. "About 30 to 40% of my women patients were sexually molested, and they retain a sense memory of being held down by the wrists while they were abused. That is now translated to being held down by the wrists while they take dictation from a lawyer in a confining cubicle. They feel trapped in the same way now as they did then."

Even something as "safe" as the deep relaxation exercises where no touch is involved and the patient is in full control (described on page 117) can be terrifying to survivors of sexual abuse. As Dr. Markison noted, it may be difficult for them to relax because of frightening imagery that arises when the body is quiet; in fact, they are often driven to hyperactivity to avoid having horrible memories arise.

If this happened to you, see a sensitive psychiatrist or psychologist to help you work through the issues surrounding sexual or physical abuse. It is also important that you are able to trust anyone who does hands-on therapy, so if you don't like that person for any reason, find someone else.

FEAR

Fear of being reinjured or becoming permanently disabled haunts RSI sufferers. This fear can sometimes trigger your symptoms, especially in the early stages of recovery, in which many people feel pain just *thinking* about using a keyboard. Their symptoms can also be triggered by seeing another RSI patient rub his hands. That usually goes away after a person advances in recovery. "There is an arbitrary and artificial distinction between mind and body," noted Dr. Rosenthal about this strong body-mind connection. "They are actually seamlessly connected."

Many RSI patients are afraid to use their hands long into recovery because they fear it will hurt. This overprotectiveness can protect you from doing too much, but after you have had plenty of time to let your body heal, *gently* test the boundaries of your pain occasionally to see if it has diminished. Maybe you will discover that opening a door didn't hurt, as you had expected. When you approach your fear, don't force things, but be curious and explore. You can always pull back if you need to.

Fear of rejection can be a problem, too. One splint-wearing man, who was not currently romantically involved, posed a question that a lot of other people probably ask themselves—namely, how will RSI affect their love lives? "Can I find a lady to sleep with who doesn't mind being scratched by Velcro?" he mused. It is common to feel vulnerable when beginning relationships, but when we are hurt or injured, it is hard to maintain self-confidence.

Worry is a subcategory of fear. Worry implies thinking, fretting, and hand-wringing, but no solution. If you're worried about losing your job, why not put the issue on hold? There is no way of predicting the future, so let yourself heal first.

Some fears are exaggerated; others aren't. Talk to your therapist to put your fears into perspective.

COPING WITH CHRONIC PAIN SYNDROME

Chronic pain syndrome is a loose term that refers to any pain that lasts longer than six months with some degree of disability. Physicians use this term for people who should be feeling better, based on the physical signs, but still have pain. At this point, the pain becomes the problem, and the doctor often doesn't know what is causing it.

People with severe chronic pain, such as reflex sympathetic dysfunction (RSD), sometimes lose their spouse—after they have already lost their jobs, homes, and health. This psychological pain, on top of the physical pain, can be devastating, so people with RSD are particularly likely candidates for psychological care. If you have serious pain, acknowledge it, but don't let it run the show.

PRIMARY AND SECONDARY GAIN

Primary and secondary gain describe unconscious processes that can occur when physical illness substitutes for direct expression of emotions. With primary gain, people experience physical symptoms instead of facing unpleasant or frightening emotions. Here is a classic example: A man gets very angry at his mother. They get in a fight, and suddenly his arm is paralyzed. The primary gain from this hysterical paralysis is that he cannot hit his mother; he has punished himself for wanting to do something he shouldn't do. The secondary gain is mother coming over and fussing over him.

Although most health-care workers say they rarely or never see secondary gain in their RSI patients, Dr. Rosenthal thinks this injury may be a last-ditch effort to put a stop to intolerable work conditions. "Getting RSI is your body's way of setting limits and saying, 'No, you can't work this hard.' If you can't choose this consciously, your body will do it for you," he said.

If this applies to you, your psychotherapist can help you understand what might be driving you to make yourself sick, and by understanding your unconscious motivation, you can learn to deal with things more directly instead of having physical ailments. This insight could pay off handsomely; for instance, you may be able to get a job in which you find self-fulfillment and control over the work pace.

KEEPING YOUR PERSPECTIVE

You can be your own best friend if you can manage to remain cheerful in spite of RSI, which is not easy. One secretary called upon her training as an actor to help her cope. "Nothing works 100%," Karen said. "If you're working for someone difficult, you're going to be angry. Accept your bad days. Maybe tomorrow will be better." Her attitude was to go on with the show. "If you've got a comedy gig and you've had a bad day, you've still got to get your laughs."

Karen kept her perspective, and thus control of the situation, by reminding herself the job wouldn't last forever and by keeping her personal goals in mind.

RSI AND OTHERS

This section deals with the interactions between the person with RSI and others. For most people, RSI is a job-related injury, and this is a problem because RSI is a hidden disability.

Dealing with Your Boss

My boss came back from the RSI lecture really determined to do something about the problem. He told me that I had to take more breaks from typing, which was fine. But he also expected me to do the same amount of work in any one day.

— Legal secretary, *Legal Business Magazine,* Jan/Feb 1992

The speaker in the above quote captures exactly the paradox facing workers with RSI: Management really seems to care about their health and wants them to get better—but it doesn't acknowledge that it will have to accept a slower pace or lighter workload—as well as the cost of retrofitting the workstation—in order to ensure that result.

Some bosses, of course, are not as nice as the one in the scenario above. One former temporary word processor, Richard, recalled an experience he had in this regard. "I was the only word processor for the whole department in an investment firm. There was an old daisy-wheel printer that made a lot of noise, and I think because people could hear that printer going all day, they expected me to produce at the same rate. I had been typing nonstop all morning, and I stood up for a second to focus my eyes on a building across the street. This guy comes up to me and says, 'Can you get this out for me?' I told him I was resting my eyes and I'd get to it as soon as I could, and he said, 'It will only take five minutes.' I said, 'Look, *I can't see.*' He just didn't get it. They all seemed to think I was a machine."

Richard's experience typifies the lack of control over work pace experienced by many lower-echelon computer operators. In the worst cases, the computer itself watches them, counting keystrokes and comparing their rate of productivity to that of their coworkers. Sometimes pay incentives are linked to high productivity, increasing the danger of overwork for the operator.

Once you have been injured, your body will never quite be the same again. The specter of reinjury hovers like a ghost, and people who think they have recovered from RSI frequently abandon their exercise, pacing, and stretch regimens only to come down with a raging relapse.

Usually, people come to respect their bodies' capacities and don't force themselves after a few relapses. Explaining to your boss why you can't work at your old pace is another story.

A woman who worked as a copywriter faced another problem common to RSI patients: skepticism. "I'm in pain all the time," she told me. "I brought it to the attention of my boss, who said, 'Oh, you just want a day off.' "

Explain RSI. One way to counter excessive demands is to educate your boss about RSI. For a quick demystification, show your boss "Common Misconceptions about RSI"(page 154). Sometimes when disbelievers see things in print they are more likely to believe it than if you told them yourself.

Delegate and Direct. Try to negotiate a lighter keyboard load with your employer. Suggest that you be in charge of supervising temporary office help. This may prove more cost-effective than hiring a replacement for you.

Be Assertive. If you don't get satisfactory results from the methods described above, use stronger measures, such as getting your doctor to go to bat for you. It is your body. No one else really knows how you feel, what your limits are, or what kind of pacing works for you.

If you feel guilty about not carrying your previous load, or if you think people suspect you of malingering, don't push yourself beyond your capacity to please them. If you do permanent damage to your muscles as a result, you will be the loser.

Your Coworkers

Your coworkers can present a problem if you have RSI and they don't. They do the same kind of work, and it doesn't bother them, so they might feel indignant that you get special treatment. Maybe they had a grudge against you to begin with; maybe they feel they are overburdened because they are pulling your load.

In any case, this can create problems for you, because if you try to resume your former pace, you are just going to reinjure yourself. Do not let guilt or pressure push you beyond your limits.

Try to explain what it is like to have RSI. Answer their questions, and say that you understand that they may feel like they have to pick up the slack for you. Encourage them not to. Show your concern: Tell them you'd hate to see them get RSI, and encourage them to take stretch breaks, too.

People can be incredibly cruel: Some RSI sufferers report being mocked when they talk about pain, teased, taunted by insensitive jokes, or made fun of when they do their exercises. Consider the source and rise above it.

"They Don't Believe Me"

If we could see into each other's souls and know the pain there, perhaps we would treat each other with kindness and consideration. But inner pain does not show, and many RSI sufferers complain that coworkers, friends, and bosses don't believe (or don't want to believe) they have a problem with their hands. If you do something that triggers pain, they might say, "Oh, come on, *that* doesn't hurt you." Or they will insist that "there's nothing wrong with your hands." *Their* hands don't hurt when they use them for minor activities, so they can't believe that yours could. Disbelievers can't see your injury, so they can't believe it could exist.

Just because there is no open wound does not mean you can't have pain, but other people may not be able to believe that. You can try to explain it to them by educating them about RSI, but if that doesn't work, don't overwork yourself for their benefit.

Tactics for Shy People

Shy, unassertive people can have an especially hard time with RSI because it means setting limits or asking others for help. One woman worked in enormous pain because she was terrified of losing her job. Another woman who should have been eligible for home care did not stand up to a state agency because she was too shy to fight for herself. Both of these women ended up losing out because they were too intimidated to stand up for themselves.

Your personality won't change overnight, so you might need to enlist the aid of your doctor or union.

One woman with carpal tunnel syndrome was at her wit's end because no one at work believed she was injured. Her doctor stepped in and said, "I can help you, I'll put you out on disability for stress; it's work-related." She did just that, and the woman got a much-needed break.

Your doctor can be your hero. See suggestions for a doctor's note on page 158.

Think about who is really pushing you, too. Is it really the boss, or is it you? "I cut productivity and speed by 50% and no one cared," said one legal word processor.

FOR THE PERMANENTLY/PARTIALLY DISABLED

If you have been permanently disabled by RSI, you may have an extra tough time. This kind of disability has a profound effect on many aspects of one's life: It can pose difficult financial and career challenges and mean major soul-searching for another identity.

For many people, self-esteem is based on what they do rather than who they are. Of course, these are interrelated, and being deprived of a career that gave you intense pleasure, self-fulfillment, and happiness can certainly be devastating. However, it doesn't mean you can't find happiness—it just won't be easy.

RSI gives us an opportunity to weigh our values. What is really important in life? Recognition for our achievements is fleeting. Money can't buy health or love. Good relationships provide a continuing source of happiness, however. So people who have serious injuries may discover deeper joys than they would have anticipated, once they figure this out.

CHANGING CAREERS

RSI is my career now.

— RSI patient

Career transitions can be tough by themselves, but if you have RSI, they are even harder. Not being able to use a computer is a major problem for many working people today. Jobs in business, finance, and law can require intensive computer use; even the UPS driver has a handheld computer. So if you cannot or will not use one, your career options can be severely limited.

In addition, the ability to use a computer almost guarantees a living wage, whereas jobs that don't require one usually don't pay well.

Some people are so eager to get away from computers they will take steep pay cuts. "If I can find something else at half the money, I will do it," said one novelist who worked as a word processor because it allowed her to devote her time to writing. Her priority was clear: She wanted to save her hands to do what she loved, even if she made less money. Other people can't envision living on less than they currently make.

Choosing a new career is a challenging, but not impossible, hurdle. If your identity depends on work, think about what you liked about your job, and then try to find other ways to feed those needs. For some people, it is collegiality; for others, it is being respected as an expert. Those good feelings can be transferred to other occupations.

Dr. Rosenthal frequently asks people this question to help them come upon something they really want to do: "If it were a perfect world, and you had all the money you needed, what would you want to do?" You certainly don't want to be "doing time" at a job you hate.

GETTING WELL TOGETHER: THE RSI SUPPORT GROUP

If we all could clap we would, but we probably shouldn't.

— Joan Lichterman, founder, East Bay RSI Support Group
(*San Francisco Examiner*, 21 March 1993)

Many RSI support groups have sprung up around the country, providing a way for people to share resources and mutual understanding of each other's plight. You can compare notes on everything from where to buy the cheapest and best office chairs to how to find a good Workers' Comp attorney. Groups can help you realize you have made progress as you see others struggle with questions you went through in an earlier phase of your recovery. Groups can offer inspiration when you see people who are worse off than you triumph over their circumstances.

Groups help because many doctors and health-care workers don't know how to deal with chronic pain, said Jewel Shuey, president and cofounder of Connecticut Chronic Pain Outreach Network. People expect support and understanding from doctors but don't get it, she explained.

People with these chronic-pain injuries look so good most of the time no one thinks there is anything wrong, Shuey added. "So if you have a good day and feel like going out, people say, 'Oh, you must be cured!'" she said. "When you have chronic pain, it doesn't get better. People don't know how to deal with that."

Your group, on the other hand, will probably know exactly what you're going through. Maybe their spouse doesn't understand, either; or their friends are tired of hearing about their troubles, too.

Groups provide an environment where people heal both themselves and others. An interesting chain reaction occurs here: When you stop focusing on your own pain and try to help others, you begin to heal yourself. You'll be important to other group members because of your ability to empathize, or because you have more experience than those who are new to RSI. Your group members will look forward to seeing you, and this will remind you of your inherent value as a person, especially if your self-esteem has been shaken by being out of work. When you feel good mentally, your body tends to feel better.

On the downside, groups have been criticized because members can seem stuck in their ruts. But if that happens, you can always find another group, or form one of your own. Or maybe you have outgrown the group or need to work in private therapy. Being in a group does not mean you might not want private therapy, too. If you can afford it, you could probably benefit from both, because each offers its own advantages.

Peer-Run Support Groups

All it takes to start a support group is two people with RSI. Jewel Shuey recommends starting small. Think of reaching one person at a time, she advises. When you forget the single person and start dealing with numbers, you lose sight of the most important purpose of the group: to provide support for people in need. Most people value small groups, because there is more intimacy and opportunity for people to share.

Shuey suggests that you do not have any affiliation with any corporation or health-care facility because people from competing institutions might not feel comfortable attending your meetings. Instead of being open to everybody, you become the "phone company group," or the "medical center group." Other institutions might not refer patients to you. In the beginning, this may not seem like a problem, but it is if you want to reach out to more than five or ten people, said Shuey. Susan Nobel, a social worker who leads an RSI group at the Mount Sinai–Irving J. Selikoff Occupational Health Clinical Center in New York, does not think it is a problem to have meetings at a health-care facility, but she does understand that people might feel reluctant to speak out if the meeting were held at the work site.

Shuey also strongly urged people not to offer to hold meetings in their homes. This creates too much stress for the facilitator to play host, and that person is probably already overworked. Instead, meet at churches, community centers, or local coffee shops during off-hours. "Some people become unbalanced because of their pain, and it's easier to handle in a neutral place," said Shuey.

Keep everything on a volunteer, free basis because many people with RSI are collecting disability and social security payments and may not be able to afford dues.

Professionally Led Support Groups

Some RSI groups are led by psychotherapists or social workers. People sometimes feel safer in such groups because, as Susan Nobel put it, "there's

---

TIPS ON STARTING AN RSI GROUP

- *Write a list of your goals.* This will help you keep focused.
- *Choose a meeting place that is centrally located and wheelchair accessible.*
- *Get a post office box.* That way you don't have to worry about people losing touch if you must change meeting locations.
- *Devise ground rules.* It is important for members to feel safe, so most groups have policies about letting only one person speak at a time and about how to handle disputes among members. Any disability can have serious implications. Be sure your members understand what confidentiality means. Read the rules before each meeting so newcomers are aware of them.
- *Start a reading list.* Books are wonderful sources of information and inspiration. You can also check the library for books on how to start a support group.
- *Put the word out.* Get a newspaper to do a story about you if you're trying to attract new members.
- *Don't do it alone.* Get a committed partner or two to share the work. Or arrange things so that the group runs itself, and the facilitator changes from time to time. This will also help prevent stagnation.

---

someone watching so no one gets wounded." A professional facilitator brings special skills to the group, such as being able to spot severe emotional disturbances that might require medication, or making sure that a shy person isn't left out. It is also easier for the facilitator to retain a sense of authority.

IF SOMEONE YOU KNOW HAS RSI

- Ask before shaking hands with people who have RSI. It may be too painful for them.
- If your hands don't hurt, do the little things for people who do have pain, such as press the elevator button, open the door, and lift the groceries. Your thoughtfulness will be truly appreciated.
- If people have symptoms of RSI, and have not been diagnosed, encourage them to see a doctor. Tell them you don't want the same thing to happen to them that happened to you. Denial is usually the first stage of RSI.

PART IV

MAINTENANCE: PREVENTING INJURY AND REINJURY

CHAPTER 14

Back to Work: From Disability to Productivity

Work is the best antidote to sorrow, my dear Watson.

— Sir Arthur Conan Doyle, *The Return of Sherlock Holmes*

Sherlock Holmes was right: Work is good for the spirit. I try to keep my patients at the job if possible, and to help them return to work as soon as possible after disability leave.

Giving advice on reentering the workplace is one of the most difficult parts of treatment. Your symptoms, emotional outlook, work situation, and recovery rate are as individual as your fingerprint, and the question of when to return to work must be decided on a case-by-case basis. There are no hard-and-fast rules about how many hours you can safely work at the keyboard once you go back. This is the point at which the work of your doctor, physical and occupational therapist, and other advisors will be put to the test. Can you really work safely? Can you employ the principles of safe technique you worked so hard to attain? Some of this will be up to you, but as you will see, a lot will also be up to your employer.

147

THE REST PERIOD

If you are severely injured, the first step toward recovery is rest. If your job requires nothing but intensive hand use, and no alternative duties can be arranged, you may need to take time off until you're better so you don't make the situation worse by continuing to stress your injured muscles.

This can take time. Even many months after you stop working, it is not unusual to experience intense residual RSI-related pain, so you may not be able to tolerate any typing at all for a while. People frequently express amazement at how the slightest computer use will trigger their symptoms after weeks or months of being away from the keyboard. "All I did was turn on the computer, list files and hit C for copy and when it was over, the underside of both my arms hurt," marvelled one woman.

Remember, though, that in this case rest does not imply completely sedentary behavior, it means avoiding strain to the injured muscles. So the rest period will actually be an active time for you: you should be faithfully following your physical therapy program and learning how to use your hands properly. Some patients at the Miller Institute gradually build their endurance during the rest period by typing for limited amounts of time each day. You can also use this time to plot your future course at work. Supervise the ergonomic improvements of your workstation during this time so everything is in place when you return to work.

Staying busy helps ward off depression and fear, so instead of worrying about your situation, try to fill your days doing all the things you wished you had the time to do before you got injured. Feeling guilty about not working won't make you heal faster, so you might as well try to enjoy yourself.

This is a great time for introspection, too: Ironically, after an enforced break from work, some people find that they don't want to go back to their old jobs at all. Their recuperation from RSI has allowed them the luxury of taking stock of their life, and some find that they want to change careers. For more on rest, see page 73.

BACK TO THE JOB

If your physical therapy has progressed to the point where you can identify and heed your body's warning signals, control pain, and pace yourself to work safely according to the guidelines on page 183, you can resume work. But you need to reenter slowly. This is one of the most difficult parts of your recovery, and deciding when it is safe for you to return to work will be one of your doctor's most difficult tasks. Be sure that your physician knows exactly what you are expected to do at work. Some employers' ideas of "light duty" are just as hard on your hands as computing, so enlist your doctor's aid if you feel you are in danger of reinjury. (See the suggestions about the doctor's note, on page 158.)

You Can't Go Back to Business as Usual

Over and over, doctors warn that injured employees cannot simply be patched up and thrown back to the same job, because they will just injure themselves all over again, only this time the injury will probably happen more quickly. Many employers have difficulty grasping this: They expect people to overwork themselves as they did before. One of the most common comments people make is, "I was fine until I went back to work. The minute I started working, the pain came back." It is absolutely essential that your doctor understand what you are required to do at work, including the pace, the workload, and your workstation setup. Your doctor may not understand what you are being required to do and would not approve if she did. Many physicians' notes saying that a person may return to light duty are not specific enough. Tell your doctor exactly what you need.

Then you need to negotiate with your employer to make your job safe. If your keyboard workload can be reduced, you might be able to do half your prior amount of keyboard work until you have your recovery under control. Look at your job. Can you delegate your keyboard work to someone else? Can you work part-time at the keyboard and spend the rest of the time doing something else? Talk to your employer and see what you can work out. If your employer balks, talk to your union official, if you have one, or enlist the aid of your doctor.

If you can work a half-day at the computer, don't do all four hours at once. Do a couple of hours in the morning and a couple in the afternoon, with lots of rest breaks. This will allow your muscles time to recover.

Some people are willing to work at noncomputer-related tasks—such as proofreading instead of word processing—until they can handle their former duties. But many patients report having trouble negotiating this kind of light duty with their employers. If this applies to you, enlist the aid of your doctor, psychiatrist, or union official and see the section in this book on the Americans With Disabilities Act (pages 196 and 207). A doctor's note stating that you need regular rest breaks and ice massage for pain can help build your case with your employer.

Plan Ahead

Sally, who worked for a major corporation, shows how assertiveness and shrewd planning can work in your favor. Before she returned to work, Sally made appropriate changes to her workstation and worked out a deal with her employers that she would only use the computer lightly, for four hours interspersed throughout the day with other duties. By vigorously standing up for herself and planning ahead, she was able to create optimum conditions for her reentry. Six months earlier, Sally had used her assertiveness to get the kind of treatment she wanted: She steadfastly refused to have surgery and obtained a second opinion for her condition. Instead of an operation, she pursued aggressive physical therapy and she did very well in recovery.

If you are shy, enlist the aid of someone to advocate for you: your doctor, union official, or attorney. But don't risk reinjury: Your employer can always replace you, but you can't replace your hands and might become unemployable if you push too hard.

Start Slowly after Vacations and Other Time Off

A lot of people are surprised to find themselves having a relapse after they come back from vacation. One woman recalled this experience: "I had been on vacation and worked my usual amount when I came back. The next morning I woke up and my hand was stiff and it was hard to type." This is like the weekend athlete syndrome: If you are sedentary during the week and then play tennis to beat the band all day Saturday, you are going to feel stiff on Sunday. So if you go away, ease back into computer work gradually, according to the pacing instructions given above.

COPING WITH WORK PRESSURES

In physical therapy and retraining, you have been trained to stop working at the first hint of pain, pace yourself carefully through your work, and perform regular stretching and strengthening exercises. It is easy enough to stick to your regimen in the safety of the doctor's office, but when you get back to the stress of work, you might be tempted to throw everything you learned out the window. Coworkers might resent your slower work pace or make cracks about your exercise breaks. A whole new set of challenges appear when you start working again.

Furthermore, management's pressure for high productivity can conflict with your ability to protect your health. It doesn't occur to managers that an employee who is recovering from RSI may never be able to return to his original productivity level, because that is what caused the injury in the first place. It is unrealistic to expect all computer operators to produce at a uniform rate, or even to expect a speedy typist to work at the same rate every day. Individual differences should be honored, and workers should be encouraged to find a comfortable pace of their own rather than being forced to keep up with the group.

Cost Cutting

In order to save money on health insurance and other benefits, employers often require employees to work longer or harder instead of hiring additional staff. Ironically, this tactic can backfire on employers; if people become injured from overtime, it causes disability and health insurance claims to skyrocket, which results in lost productivity. Many patients complain about relentless workloads; one angry young reporter with severe tennis elbow said, "There's a lot of work to be done and nobody to do it. There are days when a lot of people are out and we work extra hard."

Insensitive Management

One legal word processor, Linda, pointed out the plight of many people with RSI. "Three of us were assigned to work on one case until it was over. The first three nights we had to do straight input. We talked to our supervisor and said, 'We can't do this—we need more people or we need to alternate nights with other people so we can have an easier shift.' She refused. The only other thing we could have done was talk to the manager of the word-processing center," Linda said, but this woman was not exactly skilled in interpersonal relations. "When I was first hired, she came over to my workstation and started talking to the printer. I finally realized she was talking to me."

Linda continued in her litany of unsolved ergonomic problems. "We had a problem with glare. We tried everything: We changed the colors, tipped our screens; we wore visors," she said. In addition, "The chairs are broken—the backrests are bent the wrong way. They should support your back and they don't. The chairs are not adjustable anymore. You can either sit on the edge or lean back and try to type like that."

Linda's working conditions, unfortunately, are not uncommon—whether they reflect ignorance about the importance of ergonomics and labor relations or an unresponsive attitude of management toward personnel problems.

Peer Pressure

Peer pressure against taking breaks can be daunting, too. When I suggested to a young clerical worker that she take more rest breaks, she laughed, saying, "And they'll look at me like—!" She didn't bother to finish the sentence, but the implication was clear: Her coworkers expected her to keep up with the group, even though she was in pain. To make matters worse, this woman worked two jobs, as a clerk and grocery cashier—both of which require intensive hand use—to make ends meet. Many people depend on overtime pay or two jobs—*not* their base salary—to survive, which puts additional stress on them when they become injured.

Jobs That Present Special Problems

Temporary Word Processors

People who work as temporary word processors can have an especially difficult time. They are often called to pick up the overflow when the regular staff is swamped with work, and much of the work is expected on a rush basis. Many temporaries work 60 or more hours a week in order to nurture a career, go to school, or achieve a financial goal.

Temps also tend to work extra long hours for other reasons. For example, if they have already worked 12 hours but the work isn't finished yet, they keep going, because they fear their agency won't call them if they leave an assignment. Some temps choose to work double shifts two or three days a week so they can have the rest of their time free for their main (but perhaps low-paying) career.

So trying to do what's good for you can be daunting. One temp, Kelly, summed up the obstacles to good work practice: "The chairs have arms that get in your way, and they aren't adjustable. The monitor is bolted down so you can't adjust it. At the secretarial stations, the keyboard is on a ledge and the monitor is off to one side. There's no way to fix that," she complained.

Furthermore, Kelly thought that pacing was impracticable. "Nobody wants me to work for them unless they are terribly busy. If someone's standing over your shoulder, you don't realize that 45 minutes have gone by and you haven't had a break," Kelly continued. "I don't know what else to do. If I could do something else, I'd be doing it."

It takes a strong person to set limits with a demanding boss, especially if you fear you will be replaced for doing that. If you have an understanding boss, tell him or her that you need to take breaks from typing. Offer to do something else: Deliver a package or do some copying. Ask your agency for light assignments.

However, many temps fear that their agency will drop them if it finds out about the injury. They often work through pain because they are afraid of losing their livelihood—and are severely injured as a result. Some of my patients are deciding to take jobs that don't pay as well but keep them away from the keyboard or give them more control over pacing and work load.

Machine-Paced Jobs

If you are expected to keep pace with the computer or another person, you may not be able to keep your job. One woman became severely injured transcribing telephone calls for the deaf. She typed entire conversations, seven and a half hours a day, five or six days a week. She worked on two computers: One was for billing, the other for typing. "I'm doing the billing and typing all at the same time," she explained. "It's a high-burnout job. Some phone calls go on for hours. You couldn't tell the conversant to stop talking. One doctor estimated that I type 30,000 words an hour. I did it for two and a half years when I finally couldn't tolerate work anymore. Unless I can come back to full duty I can't come back to work." Clearly, her job was dangerous work, and unless her employer loosened its policy, she could not safely return to that job.

WORKING DURING THE RECOVERY PHASE

If you are not completely incapacitated by RSI, should you stop working? That depends. If the very sight of the keyboard makes you angry or anxious, it may be that some time off would be the best approach. Emotions such as anger or fear have a powerful effect on the body and can exacerbate symptoms (see page 136 and 138).

On the other hand, some patients' mental well-being depends on being able to work, so I look for ways to help them keep doing their jobs. If you will become severely depressed if you can't continue working, talk to your employer. Perhaps you can limit your time at the keyboard or arrange for your employer to hire someone to do your typing for you. Or maybe you can switch jobs temporarily.

TIPS FOR WORKING SAFELY

Start Slowly

The worst mistake you can make when you go back to work is to go full steam the first day. All you will get for your enthusiasm is a roaring relapse. Until patients learn to pay attention to their symptoms and pace themselves accordingly, this frustrating cycle will continue. (See the section about pacing on page 183.)

Don't Rely on Splints

Splints must be used with extreme caution, because they cause atrophy in one group of muscles and overuse in another. They can also force users to put their hands in dangerous positions. You must learn to rely on your own muscles to keep your wrists straight. If you can't type without splints, you should not be typing. (See the section about splinting on page 74.)

However, some people find that the only way to convince the boss or coworkers they have a problem is to wear a splint. If that's the case with you, leave it prominently on display, but don't work with it on.

Use Ice at Work

Most offices have refrigerators, so make some ice by filling some paper cups with water and keeping them in the freezer for pain control. Use ice massage as needed to control pain. (See the section on icing, page 96.) Icing in public signals bosses and coworkers that you are in pain, and icing is safer than splinting for that purpose.

Start an Exercise Group

A large workplace will usually have more than one injured person, so you might think of asking those people to form an exercise group. Some patients like to do their exercises together because it makes them less self-conscious than doing them alone, and they enjoy the camaraderie. Make a pact to remind your coworkers to take regular breaks or to notice if your posture or technique has deteriorated.

COMMON MISCONCEPTIONS ABOUT RSI

If you have RSI, you've probably already had one of the problems that faces everyone with it: convincing the rest of the world that despite the fact that you aren't bleeding, you are injured, and despite the fact that you're not wearing a splint, the injury will take many months to heal—much longer than the few weeks required for a broken bone.

Here are some of the most commonly asked questions about RSI. If your boss, friends, or coworkers don't understand, show them this list.

1. *I know what RSI is—that's carpal tunnel syndrome, right?*
   Wrong. The term *repetitive strain injury* covers several maladies affecting the muscles, tendons, and nerves involved in moving the hand, including deQuervain's disease, tendinitis, tenosynovitis, and carpal tunnel syndrome.

2. *I don't believe all this stuff about RSI. My aunt typed for 20 years and she never got RSI.*
   Your aunt probably used a typewriter, so she couldn't type as fast as a computer user. She also had to stop typing to change the paper, use the carriage return, and walk over to the filing cabinet instead

of retrieving a file on the screen; such variation in movement gave mini-rests to her muscles. The typewriter was steeply tiered, so she couldn't rest her wrist on the edge of the table while she worked. All of these things protected her from RSI.

3. *RSI is all in your head. People just don't want to work hard.*
That is not true. RSI is a real disease that can be diagnosed, measured, and treated. Just because you can't see the injury doesn't mean it's not there. The hardest workers are usually the first to develop RSI.

4. *I don't have to worry about repetitive strain injury—I get up and walk around.*
Although getting up and walking away from the computer is helpful, stretching your legs does nothing for RSI. You must stretch and strengthen the muscles of your neck, shoulders, and arm to protect yourself from injury.

5. *I don't type very much. I don't have to worry about getting RSI.*
Not necessarily. Repetitive strain injury is a cumulative trauma that occurs with thousands of repetitive motions over an extended period of time. So if you don't type a lot, you are probably okay—unless you do a lot of hand-intensive work such as carpentry or needlework or play a musical instrument, all of which can lead to RSI.

6. *I don't see what having long fingernails has to do with RSI.*
People with long nails tend to hold their fingers rigidly flat, contracting the muscles used to extend and flex the fingers at the same time. This co-contraction of the muscles is extremely damaging to the delicate soft tissue of the hand and forearm. Fingernails should not exceed the tip of the nail pad.

7. *I'm a big, strong man, so I won't get RSI.*
Although RSI can be related to certain hormonal imbalances or slenderness in women, RSI affects both sexes; some of the most severely injured patients are men.

8. *Smoking prevents RSI because it forces you to take breaks.*
Cigarette breaks do get people away from the keyboard, but in the long run smoking is a risk factor for RSI because nicotine constricts the blood flow. Good circulation is necessary to remove the byproducts of exertion, which can lead to buildup of scar tissue.

9. *I wear a splint when I work so I won't get RSI.*
This is not advisable, and it can be very dangerous. Wearing a splint

can allow muscles to weaken and stiffen. The use of splints should be supervised by your doctor, not self-prescribed.

10. *Once you stop working, RSI goes away.*
Unfortunately, this is generally not the case. Repetitive strain injury damages the soft tissue, which heals very slowly. The pain may go away when you stop typing, but it can return once you return to the keyboard. If you have advanced RSI, any use of the hand—such as holding a telephone or opening a door—can hurt.

11. *I have problems with my hands, but they don't hurt, so I guess I don't have RSI.*
Some dangerous forms of repetitive strain injury are painless. If you have symptoms such as clumsiness, inability to control your hands, or numbness, see your physician.

12. *Okay, so it hurts to type. You can just write everything in longhand.*
When you have RSI, any activity that involves the injured tendons and muscles can aggravate your symptoms. The act of writing can be just as painful as typing. Furthermore, simple daily activities such as using an automated teller machine or a touch-tone phone or opening doors can be excruciatingly painful for RSI sufferers.

13. *My physical therapist wants me to do all these exercises to strengthen my upper body, but I don't want to get muscular. I don't want to look unfeminine.*
Don't worry—the exercises your physical therapist prescribes won't bulk you up. These exercises will help you keep your shoulders from hunching and will tone your upper arms and shoulder blades; you will look better than ever.

14. *You should do lots of strengthening exercises if you have RSI. I do wrist curls with weights.*
Strengthening exercises must be done very carefully, and only under the supervision of a competent physician or therapist. Your muscles are weak from overuse, not underuse, and those wrist curls are causing further damage to your fragile tissue. Weights should be used only in the later stages of recovery, and they should not be handheld: They should be worn on the biceps or forearm, depending on the exercise. Strengthening exercises must be balanced with stretching, which is also crucial to prevention and recovery because it reduces the pain of RSI, reverses the injury process, and promotes healing.

15. *I'm going to get a wrist rest to prevent RSI.*
Wrist rests can't prevent RSI, and using them improperly will lead

to injury or exacerbate an existing condition. The term *wrist rest* is a misnomer. You should *never* rest your wrist while you type because it forces you to rely on the fine muscles of your hand and forearm, rather than engaging the more powerful arm and shoulder muscles to strike the key. A wrist rest should be used as a guide to keep the wrist straight: The hand should hover a half-inch above its surface. When you are thinking or *really* resting for a moment, the wrist rest provides a comfortably cushioned surface for your hands so you don't cut off circulation or damage nerves by pressing on a sharp table edge. Always use wrist rests properly.

16. *I'm going to get an ergonomic keyboard to prevent RSI.*
Before you spend hundreds of dollars on a new keyboard, you should realize that the keyboard is only one factor affecting RSI. The new keyboards have not been tested by time, so even if they seem promising now, we won't know what the outcome will be. Some of the "ergonomic" keyboards are so badly designed that they could make your RSI worse. If you have the money and want to try one, choose carefully and be sure that your physician or occupational therapist helps you adjust it correctly. Remember, though, that your keyboard cannot replace proper placement, technique, and pacing.

17. *My wrists hurt, but my physical therapist massages my neck and shoulders a lot and makes me do exercises for my upper back. She must not know what she's doing.*
On the contrary, she sounds very wise indeed. There is a good reason for working on the neck, shoulders, and back. Your physical therapist knows that the hand is strongly related to these other areas, and the hands can be the last thing to hurt when a problem begins in the neck. She needs to stretch your tight chest muscles, and your back muscles need to be strong enough to hold that open position. This allows you to improve your posture and prevent future injury.

18. *If I get injured, I'll just stop typing.*
Lots of people think RSI will go away if they stop using computers. Unfortunately, by the time RSI develops, the injury may need several months of intensive physical therapy for any improvement to occur. Not only that, by the time many people stop typing, *any* use of the hand can be difficult.

19. *I'll just let my secretary do all my typing.*
It is true that if you don't type, you will avoid computer-related RSI. But rather than "exporting" the problem by burdening your

secretary with more keyboard work—and having to wait for someone else to get something done—why not have everyone share the typing using safe keyboard technique?

20. *If I get RSI, I'll let my doctor take care of it.*
    Sorry, but your doctor can't "take care of" your RSI. Your physician can't sit up straight for you, take breaks for you, or do your exercises for you. Your recovery from RSI will depend on you.

What Should Be Included in a Doctor's Note

When your doctor writes a note for you, be sure the following items are covered:

- The note should describe your specific diagnosis.
- If you are allowed to return to work, safe working conditions should be outlined. These include the following:
  - Work requiring repetitive use of the hands and arms should be resumed gradually. Your doctor could say something like this: *I have suggested that Mr./Ms. _____ try to type for ___ hours a day with rest breaks and gradually increase the work time as his/her endurance increases. However, repetitive strain injury heals slowly and unevenly, and he/she may have varying tolerance to work on a given day. One day, he/she might be able to use the keyboard comfortably for four hours—following the pacing instructions, attached—but on another day, two hours' work may be difficult for him/her. Mr./Ms. _____ has been instructed to stop if he/she experiences pain.*
  - If possible, arrange alternative duties *that do not require use of the hand that you find painful.*
  - You should have access to ice and use it according to doctor's instructions.
  - Your workstation must be adjustable to allow for proper positioning of the body, and you must use proper typing technique.

See instructions on how to determine your tolerance level, page 183, how to ice, page 96, and how to set up your workstation, chapter 15, for more detailed information on these topics.

CHAPTER 15

Setting Up the Workstation

The best definition of ergonomics is fitting the task to the person, *not* fitting the person to the task. John Kella, a retraining coach at the Miller Institute, compares the effect of the workstation on the body to a cypress shaped by the wind. Because human beings are conforming to the workstation's unnatural demands on their bodies—and possibly because they are not in the greatest shape to begin with—most computer users wind up with rounded shoulders, concave chests, and slumped spines. If the shape of the computer conformed to the natural movements of the body, however, users might flow through movements rather than becoming rigid and tense from the constricted square grid of the computer keyboard.

It is certainly preferable to think of your hands gliding over your keyboard rather than pecking at it. However, computer and furniture design won't change overnight, so we need to make existing workstations as safe as possible until equipment is designed with human beings in mind.

THE LIMITATIONS OF ERGONOMICALLY CORRECT WORKSTATIONS

Many employers incorrectly assume that if they give their workers good equipment and well-designed workstations, they won't have a problem with RSI. The flaw in that reasoning is that work pace is not taken into consideration. When employers make ergonomic improvements, they speed up the pace of the job, observed Charley Richardson, director of the Technology and Work Program at the University of Massachusetts–Lowell. "Yet repetition is the problem, and the repetition comes out of work design, not workstation design."

Employers may offer job rotation, but if the alternate job involves the same kind of repetitive use of your hands you do now, you might as well have stayed at your old position.

Be Cautious about Buying "Ergonomic" Equipment

The explosion of computer-related RSI has spawned a booming industry in "ergonomic" furniture and health aids. Some of these accessories are valuable, but a lot of them are gimmicky, if not downright dangerous. Wrist rests are advertised to "prevent carpal tunnel syndrome" or "cut Workers' Comp claims"—things they cannot do. The photos in the catalogs show models resting their wrists on the wrist pad, a practice that leads to strain and injury. Other manufacturers sell splints and splintlike gloves that can cause or exacerbate injury. Some of these devices are even labeled "Reasonable Accommodation" (referring to the reasonable accommodation clause of the Americans With Disabilities Act)! Please be careful about buying these products. Discuss their value with your doctor or rehabilitation therapist first.

You can solve many ergonomic problems yourself inexpensively, so before you invest hundreds of dollars in new equipment, consider some of the inexpensive solutions suggested here.

THE ELEMENTS OF THE WORKSTATION

The Chair

As anyone who sits, travels on airplanes, or drives a lot knows, uncomfortable seating can make or break your disposition. At the computer, it may indirectly lead to injury by forcing you to work in awkward positions. Purchasing a good chair can make a world of difference in your comfort, and help reinforce good postural habits.

A good computer chair must adjust to support your body comfortably and correctly. If several people with disparate physical types share the same workstation, this feature becomes even more important. The seat must raise or lower so your feet are firmly planted on the floor. The seat pan should be adjustable so your pelvis tilts forward, allowing the spine to straighten. Your thighs should slope slightly toward the floor. The back rest should support your lower spine. Armrests, if you have them, should be short, so they don't bump into your desk, and padded for comfort. It is probably better not to have armrests, though, because many people use them to support their elbows when they type. You should *never* type while resting your arms on anything—the edge of the desk, the wrist rest, or the arm of the chair. If you use a backless, kneeler-type computer chair, be sure that your shins are supported so you don't strain your knees. Carry around a small tape measure so you can adjust your chair if you move from workstation to workstation. Mark the correct height for future reference.

The Desk/Keyboard Tray

Most desks are designed for writing, which makes them too high for keyboard use, so your desk should have a movable tray for your keyboard and mouse. Trays that are inset into an L-shaped desk are convenient because a higher surface for safe writing is within easy reach and you are still close to your phone and other tools.

If you don't have such a setup, it is possible to buy an add-on tray. Be sure it gives you enough adjustability, though; inches matter here. Adjust it so that your forearm is parallel to the floor when you sit with your feet flat on the ground. Measure the tray height that is proper for you and mark it so that if someone changes the height, you can easily readjust it.

The Monitor

Put the monitor directly in front of you. If you look at copy, move your copy stand from one side to the other occasionally so you are not always looking in one direction. Raise your copy holder to the same height as the monitor so you don't strain your eyes shifting back and forth from copy to screen. Some users who switch their focus from copy to screen find it comfortable to put both the copy holder and monitor directly in front of their bodies, angling them to each other as you would to display a wide-open book. This helps reduce neck tension created by holding the head turned for a long time.

Position your monitor so your eyes are level with the top of your screen. (See Figure 32.) Angle your monitor screen as you would a book unless this catches the reflection of a light. (If glare is a problem, see the section on lighting, page 163.)

FIGURE 32   How To Set Up Your Workstation.
(Copyright 1992 Time Inc. Reprinted by permission.)

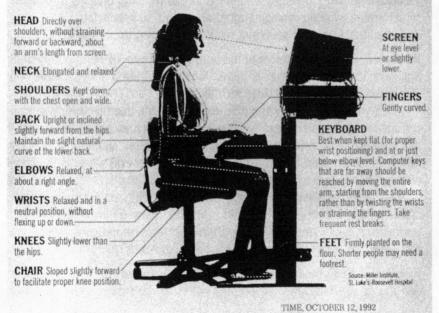

HEAD Directly over shoulders, without straining forward or backward, about an arm's length from screen.

NECK Elongated and relaxed.

SHOULDERS Kept down, with the chest open and wide.

BACK Upright or inclined slightly forward from the hips. Maintain the slight natural curve of the lower back.

ELBOWS Relaxed, at about a right angle.

WRISTS Relaxed and in a neutral position, without flexing up or down.

KNEES Slightly lower than the hips.

CHAIR Sloped slightly forward to facilitate proper knee position.

SCREEN At eye level or slightly lower.

FINGERS Gently curved.

KEYBOARD Best when kept flat (for proper wrist positioning) and at or just below elbow level. Computer keys that are far away should be reached by moving the entire arm, starting from the shoulders, rather than by twisting the wrists or straining the fingers. Take frequent rest breaks.

FEET Firmly planted on the floor. Shorter people may need a footrest.

Source: Miller Institute, St. Luke's-Roosevelt Hospital

TIME, OCTOBER 12, 1992

It is very important that you don't place your monitor too high. In order to compensate for this angle, you will tilt your head back to look up at the screen. This knocks your neck out of alignment and causes headache. Think of the head as a bowling ball balanced atop the spine. If it sits in perfect alignment, with the ears in line with the shoulders, it requires little muscular support. If you pitch your head forward, your neck muscles—which are relatively weak—must strain to support its weight.

Colors. Colors per se have not proven to be a significant factor in visual safety, and so they can be your own choice. A pale blue or grey background with dark letters reduces glare and has a soothing effect. Easy readability and clarity are the keys to comfort. Avoid color combinations that are difficult to tell apart.

Some people still use old-fashioned green monitors. If you see pink after-images (the McCullough effect, an apparently harmless phenomenon) after you've looked at a green screen all day, either buy a new monitor or turn down the brightness of your screen.

Contrast. With contrast, easy readability should be your guide. Adjust your controls until characters are crisp and sharp.

Flicker. What you see on your screen is created by an electronic beam that "paints" the image repeatedly. This "refresh rate" results in flickering, which most computer users do not perceive, but which nonetheless contributes to eyestrain and headaches. The most common refresh rate is 60 times per second or greater. Currently, not enough is known about the effects of flicker to determine whether changing monitors would be beneficial.

If the flicker on your screen is visible, turn down the brightness.

Resolution. Resolution refers to the number of pixels (or dots) per inch on a screen. In general, denser is better. Smaller dot pitch is better, too. You will probably pay a higher price for this feature.

When you are buying a monitor, don't go by the manufacturer's specifications alone, because these won't tell you as much as seeing the monitor in action with your own eyes. Go to the computer store and look at as many monitors as you can. Look at the same word on several screens. Which is crisper? Which one would you prefer to look at all day?

Look at the edges of the screen, because warping and fuzziness will be more apparent there. Get a monitor with as many controls as you can, because you may prefer taller or shorter letters, or more or less space between lines. You want sharp contrast and easy readability.

Polarity. Display polarity is the relationship between the text characters and the background. *Positive polarity* refers to dark characters on a light background (like a page from a book); *negative polarity* is white or light characters on a dark screen (like DOS).

Positive polarity is best. The eye is trained to work with positive polarity, because almost everything you read—books, newspapers, and letters—is presented in that format. In addition, if you work from copy, your pupils won't have to dilate and constrict constantly as you move from page to screen. Screens with a light background will present fewer problems with glare as well.

Lighting

The lighting designer trying to meet every office worker's preferences has a tough job indeed! Good lighting is crucial for comfort, but lighting needs can vary drastically from person to person. Older people need more light to see clearly than younger people. Some people are extremely sensitive to light; others don't seem to notice. Some people love dim rooms and detest bright lights; others hate such cavelike environs.

In addition to personal tastes and needs, the computer itself presents complications. Because the monitor is a lamp (internally lit), you don't need to shine light on the computer screen. If you find you need more light to illuminate the copy, get a small reading lamp and focus it on the copyholder. Because the monitor also acts as a mirror (reflecting objects and light), be careful to position it away from glare. Ideally, there should be plenty of soft light to illuminate the copy stand and desk surface, but no light source should reflect from the screen.

Sunlight streaming through a window may seem like a beautiful image, but it is not helpful if you work with a computer. Light from both natural and artificial sources can bounce off your screen and cause annoying glare, which can result in eyestrain. Your body may also unconsciously assume a cramped position to compensate for glare, and you will pay for this awkward posture with muscle pain.

To avoid glare, you must look for several culprits: windows; overhead lighting fixtures; and bright, reflective surfaces such as desk surfaces, highly polished floors, or even your own jewelry. To find a good position for your monitor, turn the screen off and look for a reflection, or experiment with a large handheld mirror so you don't have to do a lot of heavy lifting. Make sure that no bright light enters your sight lines as you gaze at the screen. Try to put your monitor perpendicular to the window and between rows of overhead lights. Tilt the screen to reduce reflections from light sources behind you.

If you can't move your VDT, either buy or make a hood out of cardboard and tape it to the monitor to shield the screen from light sources. As a last resort, you can also get antiglare filters that fit directly on the screen. Some of these filters make it hard to see the characters, so use them only if the other measures fail, and be sure to try different models before buying one so you can find one that doesn't fatigue your eyes.

Because the angle of the sun changes as the earth rotates, window coverings should be adjustable. Vertical blinds are nice because they can be angled to block light but still allow another person to see the view. Overhead lighting fixtures should be perpendicular to the screen.

A dirty screen can also increase glare. Get into the habit of dusting it every day. Don't use your hands for this; use screen wipes. The dust from the monitor is electromagnetically charged, and if you touch your face with it, it can cause skin problems.

The Keyboard

The QWERTY Keyboard. The standard QWERTY keyboard (so named because of the arrangement of the top row of letters) is riddled with design flaws. It forces the user to use an unnatural and stressful palms-down position (pronation), which not everyone can do comfortably. According to Robert Markison, 15% of humans are not fit for sustained pronation because of their anatomy. Commonly used keys, such as the A and the Shift keys, are traditionally struck with the pinkie, the weakest finger in the hand. The placement of the number pad and important function keys on the right side forces the overuse of the right hand, which can cause great dismay to people who are right-handed. Certain keyboards have rows of function keys, which usually require the Shift, Alt, or Control key to be held down. Rather than use two hands to accomplish this, people stretch the fingers of one hand, which strains the tendons. Because most people don't know any better, they twist their hands to the outside (ulnar deviation), which puts stress on the tendons (see Figure 33).

Furthermore, the kickstand tilts the keyboard the wrong way, causing users to work in a dorsiflexed position (wrists bent upward as though to push open a door), which is worsened by most users' tendency to rest their wrists on the edge of the desk while they work. (See Figure 1 on page 16). Because people erroneously assume that the kickstand is angled the correct way, many users hike it up as high as it will go!

Manual typewriter keys had a springy feel, so users could sense when they were coming to the end of the keystroke and adjust the amount of force they used. Computer keys often don't have any cushion at all, so your fingers do the equivalent of crashing into concrete, which is particularly problematic for people who tend to use too much force anyway. One young

FIGURE 33 Ulnar Deviation at the Keyboard.
The wrists are bent sideways to reach keys, straining the tendons in the hand and forearm.

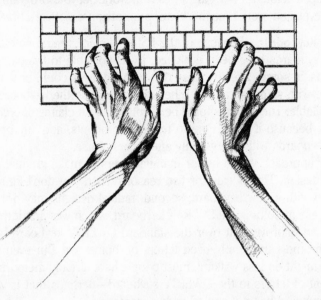

man complained of intense sensitivity at the ends of all his fingers, and pain, numbness, and tingling in his fingertips and the joints of his hands. He was in very good shape and had no other sign of RSI-related damage, but he was a "clacker," and all that pounding had made his fingers supersensitive. His problem was compounded by his keyboard, which he described as "brittle."

Given its current inadequacies, it is no wonder that the inanimate keyboard often becomes a lightning rod for patients' anger. People can become so enraged by their injury that they feel like hurling their keyboard out the window. One woman declared she was allergic to the keyboard and refused to go near it during a retraining session!

However, it is unfair to ascribe the entire burden of RSI to the design of the keyboard, faulty as it is. Even the QWERTY keyboard can be used safely if you know how, whereas some of the much-touted new ergonomic designs can actually increase the likelihood of developing RSI if they are improperly used.

Use Hot Keys, Macros, and Save. Save keystrokes by taking advantage of hot keys and macros. Some programs, which act as the shift-lock, make keys "sticky," and allow users to make two-keystroke motions with one hand.

You should also program your computer to prompt you to take breaks. Some people find it helpful to personalize their prompt with messages such as

"Breathe," "Do your eye exercises," "Stretch," or "Relax." If you don't have the capability to do that, many computer programs allow you to decide how many minutes elapse before the software saves your work. Set your program to your tolerance level, and every time the "Save" prompt appears, take a break.

Ergonomic Keyboards. Because of the RSI epidemic, several so-called ergonomic keyboards have been designed. I was not able to evaluate all the new designs, in some cases because the manufacturers could or would not provide me with samples, and in other cases because the keyboards were not yet available. The public should be skeptical about claims of ergonomic superiority, because it takes time to test new products, and any problems with the keyboards will emerge only after years of use.

A better approach would be for manufacturers to make gradual modifications in design. This is true for two reasons: First, you don't know what will happen with a new keyboard; second, radical designs may not be accepted. A case in point is the DVORAK keyboard, which was first introduced in 1932 as an improvement over the standard QWERTY keyboard because it places the most frequently used letters on home row. But even though the fingers might do less walking, most people have already memorized the arrangement of letters in the QWERTY keyboard—perhaps that is why the DVORAK keyboard has not gained wide acceptance.

If you want to try the DVORAK, however, you can easily convert your QWERTY keyboard by reconfiguring your software and changing the keycaps.

Many designers lack a solid understanding of anatomy and knowledge of how the body is meant to move. Some manufacturers have the misguided notion that the answer to RSI is to essentially immobilize the hand by making it do as little as possible. This approach is mistaken; the tendons and muscles of the entire upper extremity (hand, forearm, and shoulder) should move freely and effortlessly in a coordinated way, *not* be held in a rigidly static position. One new keyboard, for instance, could be quite dangerous because it not only restricts finger movement, but also automatically puts the hand in dorsiflexion and ulnar deviation—a deadly double-whammy.

Other keyboards allow a less strained position of the hand (they either are split in two parts or rise in the middle like a pyramid). These keyboards also have a great deal of adjustability, but this is a two-edged sword: They have potential to relieve extrinsic ergonomic problems, but unless they are properly adjusted, you can get into a harmful position with them. They should be fitted to the individual by a knowledgeable person.

These keyboards are too new for anyone to know whether they will be safer over the long term. Even if some of the new keyboards prove to be safe, remember that keyboard design will never substitute for retraining, good posture, and proper positioning.

Mice and Trackballs. An explosion of mouselike devices has hit the computer market, which presents a dilemma for computer users. My coauthor and I tried to evaluate as many as we could for this book, and the result of our effort will interest you. We couldn't find a single mouse or trackball we felt was safe to use for extended periods of time. Worse, we had the same problem you will probably have if you try to buy one: Most of the stores kept the devices wrapped in their sealed boxes and refused to take them out so we could hold them or see how they worked. The photographs on the packages did not clearly show how the device should be operated, either. Consumers are expected to buy them on blind faith. We don't recommend buying any handheld tool you haven't tried first. You can get around this problem by ordering these devices from mail-order catalogs that guarantee your money back if you aren't satisfied.

A lot of study has been focused on the keyboard, but little on these accessories. However, judging from their design, I doubt they were built for hand safety: Mice inherently strain the hand by forcing repetitive use of one digit, and they are awkward to hold. Not only that, the orientation always has to be vertical in order to get the cursor to move the right way. Some of the most serious injuries I have seen have come from mouse use. See page 182 for mouse technique.

Trackballs also present problems, because even though you can click on and move the cursor instead of dragging—and thus avoid gripping—they sometimes rely on one or two digits of one hand and encourage excessive and awkward wrist or thumb motion. Styluses pose problems for the same reasons ordinary pen does: If people hold them in a death grip, it can lead to writer's cramp, a very serious injury. (See the section on focal dystonia, page 59.) If you use a stylus, try a pen expander (see page 171 and 183).

New devices that "read" handwriting input with an electronic stylus are coming on the market, too. If you use one of these, be sure to see the information in Chapter 16 on how to hold a pen.

All of these input devices need long-term studies to determine whether they are safe to use.

Laptops. Laptop computers are pitched as a wonderful boon for people who want to work on airplanes, in hotels, or in other places where personal or mainframe computers are unavailable. They have become quite sophisticated since the first models appeared, and some now even have built-in printers.

People with RSI should use laptops with extreme caution, however. First of all, the keyboard and screen may not be detachable, forcing awkward hand and head positions. Some of the screens can be hard on the eyes because of the shadowy trail of afterimages left on the screen. They are also quite heavy to carry, especially once you add the power pack, your briefcase, and reference materials.

If you have RSI, think twice before investing in a laptop. Is this work really so urgent it can't wait until you can get to a desk with a proper ergonomic setup? It is virtually impossible to work comfortably from the constrained space on a plane or train, or the makeshift furniture in your hotel room. Laptops feed into our society's incessant drive to work, which is a primary risk factor for RSI.

If you must use a laptop, try to position it as well as you can, and take more breaks than usual if you are forced into awkward positioning. Be sure to choose the highest-quality screen in order to avoid eyestrain.

Voice-Activated Computers.   A number of people who can't use their hands use voice-activated computers. Although this new technology can be a boon to someone disabled by RSI, it cannot be viewed as a panacea, because it can endanger another body part: the vocal folds (which most people call vocal cords).

Talking all day is tough work, and talking and sitting can be a dangerous combination. New York City speech/language pathologist John Haskell notes that when people sit, they don't use the same energy they would if they were standing. Rather, they tend to use a lower pitch, restrict the variety of tone, and breathe shallowly.

People who use voice-activated computers will have to view themselves as vocal athletes to survive the strain to their vocal apparatus. "The voice is their instrument, and it has to be healthy," says Dr. Haskell. He advises drinking plenty of water to keep the throat lubricated and taking frequent rest breaks (every 30 minutes or so). "Approach work like a radio broadcaster," he suggested. Speak to the computer as though you were talking to a person—with animation and projection—rather than a flat monotone. Though this may be difficult to do if you are reading boring data, try, because the voice operates best when it is natural and conversational.

The working environment could present another possible problem with voice-activated computers: If people don't have private booths, they might speak softly out of self-consciousness, which can strain the voice. If you work all day with your voice, you will also have to be careful how you use it when you are not working. Don't smoke anything; avoid smoky or dusty environments; and see an ear, nose, and throat specialist if you experience problems such as persistent hoarseness or a sore throat. You may also benefit from speech training to learn how to use your voice without straining it.

SPECIAL SITUATIONS
Typing Standing Up

If you work standing up, as do clerks at car-rental agencies, you are at special risk, because you will certainly be working in dorsiflexion unless the counter is high enough for you. Be sure you do enough stretching and strengthening exercises to counteract this poor setup. Better yet, ask your employer to make safe adjustments to your workstation.

The Future

With amazing new technology advances dazzling the public frequently, some people joke that we will all have small computers implanted in our wrists in the future. That day may never come, but there are prototype computers that read "thought waves" through electrodes attached to the scalp. Touch-activated screens are already commonly used for automatic teller devices. Scanners that "read" handwriting are also available. Computers are responding to voice commands. We hope the engineers who create these devices will think of the user's safety and comfort, rather than merely boosting productivity.

REST ACCESSORIES
Wrist Rests

I call wrist rests "wrist guides" because that's what they should do: guide your wrists to keep them straight. Most people do what the misnomer implies and rest their wrists on them, which leads to increased strain and injury.

You should never rest your wrists while you work; rather, let them hover a half-inch above the wrist rest (see Figure 35 on page 178). Take frequent mini-breaks (see page 184 for instructions) and rest your wrists when you're not typing.

Almost no one positions the keyboard correctly. First, flatten the kickstand and put a three-quarter-inch support under the keyboard so it slopes down, not up, from the fingers. Then raise the near end of the keyboard so the space bar is level with the top of the wrist rest. Paper clip boxes and door wedges work fine; just tape them down so they don't move (see Figure 35 on page 178.) Make sure you are able to lower your table to the proper height if you use this setup.

Elbow Rests

Elbow rests are not to be confused with the arm rests of a chair. Elbow rests are movable stirrups designed to support your forearm while you work. Using an elbow rest is like trying to run a marathon on crutches. I don't like them because they actually encourage RSI by forcing the small muscles of the hand to do the work instead of letting the arm carry the hand. This leads to muscle tightening and atrophy. In *extremely rare* cases, we use elbow rests during retraining, rather like training wheels on a bicycle. But you should never rest your elbows while you work. The pressure can cause nerve damage and it puts enormous strain on the finger tendons. It is better to rest your elbow on your armrests occasionally *when you are not typing*.

Footrests

You don't need a footrest if you can place your feet on the floor and still have your forearms in good position. If your feet dangle, put a stable object beneath your feet so that you are positioned correctly.

Some people like ergonomic footrests that allow the feet to move forward and back. Other people find it a nuisance to have something under their feet, especially if they get up and down frequently and find themselves tripping over their footrests. If you find it comfortable, use it correctly. Don't allow your knees to be higher than your hips—it strains your spine.

Helpful Tools

Scanners

Scanners are a godsend to anyone with RSI, because instead of having to type new input, you can just scan prepared text into the computer and save your hands for editing.

Telephone Headsets

One of the most common sights in any home, office, or phone booth is people holding the receiver with their shoulder while their hands do something else. This is a very bad habit, because when you hold the phone with your upraised shoulder, you not only severely tense and strain the neck muscles and compress the nerves at the neck; you also force your wrists into ulnar deviation because you have to hold your upper arm close to your ribs to keep the phone in place. People who type and talk on a handset risk severe injury to the neck, shoulders, wrist, and forearm. (See the phone shoulder discussion, page 53.)

If you don't believe your phone style can damage your body, consider the case of a young newsman. He came to the office in severe pain from habitually holding the phone with his shoulder while he typed. He was 32 years old, but his X rays looked like they belonged to a 72-year-old. An MRI showed spinal cord compression from a herniated disk. He was out of work for months and might always have problems from arthritis.

Get a headset if you spend a lot of time on the phone while you type. Light ones such as the ones used by telephone operators are nice. Otherwise, don't type and talk at the same time.

Copyholders

Copyholders should be placed at the same level as your monitor so your eyes don't have to constantly refocus as you switch from page to screen. Be sure you don't have to crane your neck to see the copy. Switch the copyholder from left to right of the monitor regularly—or have one on each side—to balance the use of your neck muscles.

Don't get rigid about things, though. When we told one newspaper reporter how to position his copy, he said, "In real life, when I'm on deadline, I'm working from 17 different pieces of paper, and I'm looking all over the place. It's impossible for me to do that."

This reporter saved himself from the possible strain of his awkward positioning because he worked out with weights several times a week and kept his neck muscles stretched and supple. If you find yourself working in strained positions occasionally, remember to undo the potential damage by stretching frequently and staying in good shape.

Pen Expanders

If you find it difficult to write with a thin pen, or if you tend to grip your pen too tightly, get a pen expander from your stationer. These are made from either plastic or foam rubber and cost under a dollar. By expanding the circumference of the pen, they allow your fingers to work in a more relaxed position and reduce the strain of handwriting. Foam hair-curlers also work.

It is also helpful to use soft-lead pencils and pens that require a light touch, and felt-tip or roller balls rather than ballpoint pens, so you don't have to use pressure to write. Weighted pens are also available for people who have trouble pressing. (See the Resources section, page 209.)

Timers

If you can program your computer to prompt you to take a break, do so. If not, use a wristwatch or kitchen timer to remind you to take your stretch breaks. Generally speaking, a 5- to 10-minute break for every 25 minutes at the keyboard is a good maintenance level. If you have been injured and are coming back to work slowly, find your tolerance level and set the timer accordingly. (See the section on pacing, page 183.)

Mirrors

Mirrors can be extremely useful—and cheap—feedback tools. If you position one on your workstation, you will be able to see if you are keeping your spine and neck in alignment and your shoulders open and relaxed; if your face looks drawn, you will know that it's time for a break. Mirrors are also useful for learning the retraining techniques described in Chapter 16.

CHEAP MODIFICATIONS

Modifying your workstation doesn't need to cost a fortune (to the tune of an average of $1,500 per workstation!), and I've seen some gizmos that would make me laugh if it weren't for the outrageous claims and hefty price tag attached to them. Computers are packed in high-quality, soft foam that can easily be cut into pelvic tilt cushion or lumbar rolls to support your lower back. Rolled-up towels or pillows can serve the same purpose in a pinch. You can make your own wrist rest or mouse pad with foam rubber. (Make it three inches deep, the length of your keyboard, and the height of your space bar.) Foam hair-curlers work as pen, utensil, and tool adapters.

Telephone books or reams of paper can be used to raise your terminal to a better height. Cardboard can shield your monitor from glare. If you have a handy friend, prevail upon him or her to build you an adjustable table tray. Use your imagination.

If your keyboard has little give, put a piece of thin foam under your keyboard to cushion the keystroke, or put foam on the keys themselves (use earring cushions or corn pads with holes in the middle so you can still read the keys).

DON'T BE A SUCKER

Don't buy keyboards (which we saw priced from $100 to $1,200) or gimmicky devices or accessories unless you are positive they are worth the cost—and preferably have been evaluated by a competent doctor or occupational therapist. Don't be taken in by slick advertising that won't deliver. Don't buy a chair you haven't sat on. If you order from catalogs, make sure there is a money-back guarantee.

TROUBLESHOOTING FOR RSI

RSI is a baffling disease, with symptoms coming and going, or surfacing in new places. Puzzling as it seems, you can usually find a reason for pain, if you think about it long enough. One of the first questions your rehabilitation

TROUBLESHOOTING FOR PAIN

Problem	Possible Cause	Try This
Frequent headaches, eyestrain, or other vision problems	Need corrective lenses or new prescription	Consult eye doctor
Pain on one side of neck	Monitor to the side	Move monitor in front of you
	Vision problem that causes head-tilting	Have vision checked by competent eye doctor
Overall neck pain	Chin juts forward while seated	Postural retraining; supervised neck exercises; massage
Headaches; pain in neck	Screen too high	Lower screen
	Bifocals not corrected for computer work	Get new prescription for VDT work
	Muscle tension	Relaxation and supervised stretching exercises
Pain in neck and shoulder on one side	Typing while holding telephone receiver between neck and shoulder	Use a headset
Pain in shoulder	Poor conditioning; tension; concave posture	Stretching exercises; range of motion exercises for shoulder and front of chest; massage
Pain in upper back	Poor conditioning; poor posture; tension; poor seating	Postural retraining; stretching and strengthening exercises; massage; better chair
Pain in elbow	Keyboard raised in back (see Figure 1 on page 16); table too high; overuse	Raise front of keyboard (see Figure 35 on page 178); lower table; take frequent breaks; slow down; technique retraining; stretching and strengthening exercises
Numbness, pain in elbow	Leaning on elbow; keyboard too high	Stop leaning on elbow; lower table

Pain on top of forearm along pinkie side	Ulnar deviation; little finger held aloft as you work; flat-fingered typing	Technique retraining; keep fingernails short
Pain on bottom of forearm	Overuse; dorsiflexion; hands dropped from wrist (flexed)	Breaks; technique retraining; stretching; massage
Numbness in fingers; pain in wrists	Dorsiflexion; resting wrists on edge of desk or wrist rest while you type; edge of desk cutting into wrist	Technique retraining; don't rest wrists while typing
Pain in thumb or thumb-side of wrist	Holding thumb up while typing; hitting space bar too hard; overuse	Technique retraining; use fingers instead of thumb for space-bar; rest breaks
Pain in fingertips	Pounding keyboard	Technique retraining; use a light touch
Lower back pain	Poor conditioning; poor posture; slouching in seat; weak muscles; sitting with one foot under buttocks; poor seating	Postural retraining; lumbar roll cushion to support lower back; stretching and strengthening exercises; stop sitting on calves or feet; better chair with adjustable seat pan or pelvic tilt cushion
Numbness in legs	Seat pan cuts off circulation; feet dangle; sitting with one foot under buttocks	Tilt seat pan; get footrest if feet don't rest flat on floor; stop sitting on legs or feet

therapist will probably ask you when you complain of symptoms is, "What were you doing to cause it?"

The troubleshooting guide is intended to help you track down sources of pain. Remember, though, that the human body operates in mysterious ways. No one fully understands pain or other symptoms; sometimes things seem to happen for no reason at all. These suggestions are not meant to replace a medical examination. If they don't help quickly, see a doctor: You may have a problem that is not related to your workstation setup.

Remember, many of these symptoms could be related to serious underlying disease. If they persist, see a physician.

CHAPTER 16

Typing Technique Retraining for Computer Athletes

Typing technique is the ignored stepchild of ergonomics. Technique refers to how you hold your hands when you strike the keys, how much force you use, and how you move your hands and arms over the keyboard. If you have RSI, you can improve your posture, get the best ergonomic furniture money can buy, take breaks, and keep your upper body in good shape, but if you persist in using bad technique, you will be plagued with relapses. If you don't have RSI, using bad technique is a good way to get it. Unlike extrinsic factors that cause RSI, such as your workstation design, damage caused by technique is intrinsic, that is, it depends on how you use your hands. Certainly, it is a lot easier to adjust your furniture than modify deeply ingrained movements of your body.

Virtually all the people we see have unwittingly contributed to RSI by using poor technique at the keyboard. If you hit your thumb with a hammer, you would get a bruise that would heal and eventually go away—unless you kept hitting yourself. So when you hold your hands improperly, you essentially assault your own body with every keystroke. Until the offending behavior stops, RSI will continue.

You wouldn't expect a person to sit down at a piano and play a piece by Mozart without training. In the same way, computer users need to learn good technique, but this is not instinctive; in fact, it is counterintuitive. That is why we retrain every patient on proper keyboard technique to stop the cycle of injury and reinjury. Ideally, though, people should learn these techniques from the beginning to avoid RSI entirely.

THE ORIGINS OF RETRAINING

I founded the Miller Institute for Performing Artists in 1985 to help injured dancers, singers, and musicians keep working. Musicians' hands take similar punishment to those of computer operators because of rigorous performance, rehearsal, and audition schedules. If they love what they do, RSI is both a heartbreaker and a career wrecker. Bad technique can kill careers, and we wanted to discover ways to allow the musicians to keep performing—safely.

To study their problems, our team videotaped over 750 performers at work. When we analyzed the tapes, we noticed that their injuries were connected to the shape of their instruments and the way they played (their technique). So we made subtle adjustments to their playing style, showing them how to avoid dangerous positions such as dorsiflexion and ulnar deviation. We also designed modifications for their instruments, so a flutist with a short pinkie finger wouldn't have to reach as far for the stop, for instance. We have helped hundreds of musicians to break habits that were injuring them, particularly performers afflicted with focal dystonia.

Based on our experience with musicians, we were able to develop a safe typing technique for computer operators when they started appearing at the Institute a few years ago.

YOU ARE A COMPUTER ATHLETE

Computing is a sport in a way, and the importance of technique retraining cannot be overemphasized. If you work improperly, you will keep reinjuring yourself, and RSI will become chronic. Numerous analogies can be made to other athletic endeavors: Runners who let their feet turn out when they run get knee problems; ballet dancers who don't stretch their calves get Achilles tendinitis; tennis players who use bad form get elbow problems. You must prevent injuries with good technique.

Many users habitually use the keyboard much longer than any smart athlete would. Runners don't run eight-hour marathons every day, yet people think nothing of spending eight hours or more a day at the keyboard. Hockey teams take two days off a week, weight lifters rest certain muscles every other day—yet computer users often work overtime, day after day, under stressful conditions, without even taking regular breaks! The fact that you are sitting down reinforces the misconception that you are resting, when in fact your hands are being subjected to intense stress.

One of the most popular misconceptions about computer work is that it is an "easy" activity, when in fact it is quite strenuous for your hands and arms. People wonder how the keyboard, which has a such a light touch, could be dangerous. But it is precisely this feature that allows great speed, thus great repetition of hundreds of thousands of keystrokes a day, and leads to RSI.

But even though computing works your hands and forearms, it is still a sedentary activity, so don't get the idea that it replaces an overall fitness program. You need to consistently follow an exercise routine that involves aerobic activity in addition to keeping your upper body lithe and strong to stay in shape for the keyboard.

BASIC TYPING TECHNIQUE TO PREVENT RSI

Keep Your Wrist Straight

News articles on RSI often say that it is important to keep the wrist straight while typing. But as you will see, this idea needs to be fully understood in order to be employed. Some people think they are keeping their wrist straight when they are actually ulnar deviating (moving the hands sideways from the wrist to the outside with windshield wiper motion as in Figure 32). For the wrist to be neutral, it must be parallel to the floor and the middle finger must be at the center of the wrist. (See Figure 3 on page 17, Figure 35 on page 178, and Figure 34, below.)

Exercise to Find the Angle Where
Your Forearm Is Parallel to the Floor

Stand or sit sideways in front of a full-length mirror and bend your forearms until you form a 90-degree angle at your elbow. Keep your middle finger in line with your wrist. Do this as often as it takes

FIGURE 34   Neutral Position at the Keyboard.
Here the middle knuckle is aligned with the center of the wrist, and the arm moves the hand over the keyboard along the lines of a chevron rather than stretching fingers to reach the keys.

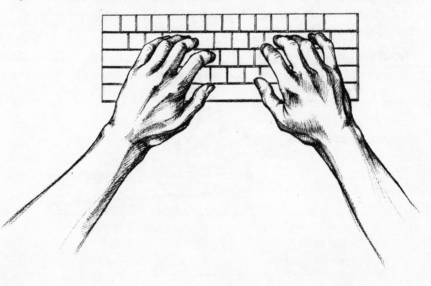

to remember that feeling within your own body. Remember, your table height must accommodate this position, so either raise your chair or buy a slide-out tray for the keyboard to get the proper height. (See page 160.) Be sure to move your chair close enough in to the keyboard that you can relax your upper arms at your side rather than reaching out for the keyboard.

Don't Rest Your Wrists While You Type

The most common postural mistake people make is resting their wrists, elbows, or forearms on the edge of the desk or the wrist rest while they type (as in Figure 1 on page 16). It seems easier to them, but it actually is not. You wouldn't throw a baseball very far if you threw from the wrist alone because you wouldn't have any power. It is like trying to walk using only your feet, without involving your hips or knees; you are making all the little muscles and tendons do the work the big muscles should be doing, and you are asking for trouble.

When you type, let your wrists float above the wrist rest as in Figure 35. Rest your wrists *only* while you aren't typing.

Exercise to Gain Awareness of Moving the Whole Arm

Follow the steps in the previous exercise to find neutral wrist position. Holding your hands suspended over the keyboard, make a few circles in the air just over the keys. Let the strong muscle of the back, shoulders, and forearms position your hands, allowing the fingers to move lightly from an unstressed position. Instead of resting your hands, get used to using your whole arm to move your hands over the keys.

FIGURE 35 Proper Wrist Angle.

For a description of this keyboard setup, see page 169.

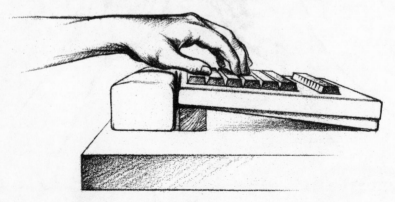

TIP: **1.** If you catch yourself resting your wrists or forearms on your wrist-pad, pretend that it is hot or has sharp prongs on it. Don't get lazy with this—resting is very damaging to your tendons.

2. To prevent ulnar deviation, think of moving your hands (wrists neutral) inward along the lines of an inverted V. (See Figure 34 on page 177.) Some of the new ergonomic keyboard designs have made maintaining a neutral wrist position easier by splitting the keyboard.

Avoid Stretching the Fingers to Reach Faraway Keys

Don't stretch for faraway keys (such as Escape, End, Insert and Delete, or the number pad); move your arm from the shoulder, position your fingers over the key, and *then* strike. Keep the hand in proper alignment while striking. This means no ulnar or radial deviation (twisting the hand to the side so the middle finger is no longer in line with the center of the wrist). See Figure 34 on page 177 for an example of proper positioning.

Exercise to Avoid Stretching Fingers

Hold your hands over home row (this row contains the letters AS-DFG). Then move your whole hand over to the number pad and strike a key. Go back to home row. Then move your whole hand up to one of the function keys and strike a key. Continue until you are accustomed to moving your hand as a unit instead of stretching your fingers.

TIP: Center the portion of the keyboard you use the most directly in front of your body. If you type copy, for instance, the G and H should be approximately in line with your navel. If you use the number pad most often, center it directly in front of your typing hand so that the middle finger stays in the center of the wrist and the forearm is straight. In this case, the right Alt or Enter key will be in front of your navel.

FIST TRICK

If you want to give your hands a break from the stressful palms-down position and are not doing something that requires speed, hold a fat marker or blunt-capped pen in your fist as though you were going to pound on the table or hold a vertical bus pole. Now touch the computer keys with your marker or pen. This puts your hand, wrist, and forearm in an unstrained position. Remember not to grip your pen.

Keep Fingers Curved

Typing with thumbs and pinkies upraised is another common problem among computer typists. Some people hold their thumbs in the air for fear they will accidently hit the space bar; others have what I call the "Buckingham Palace syndrome"—that is, they hold their pinkies aloft as though they were drinking tea.

Both habits will land you in a whole lot of trouble. If you hold your thumb rigid, you are likely to give yourself tendinitis of the thumb (deQuervain's disease). If you hold your pinkie up, your forearm's muscles will be strained. Both conditions can be quite painful and debilitating.

Exercise to Keep Your Fingers Curved

Let your hands drop to your sides, as in the first exercise. Your fingers will be naturally curved. Keeping this relaxed position, bring your hands to the keyboard. Your forearms should be parallel to the floor, with your middle finger in line with the center of your wrist. Your fingers should be curved so that you strike the keys with the fingertips. Don't rest your wrist; let the hand remain poised in the air with fingers effortlessly curved. This is the way you should hold them when you type.

Relax the Thumb

Learning to relax the thumb is particularly difficult. Let it rest as much as possible to counteract this tendency. By relaxing the thumb, you tend to relax the rest of the hand.

Exercise to Learn to Relax the Thumb

Rest your hand palm down on the table. Consciously lift your thumb, and then let it drop. Pay attention to what both sensations feel like. If you catch yourself tensing your thumb, let the thumb rest. Keep doing that until it becomes second nature to you.

TIP: **1.** If you point your thumb or pinkie, try putting a piece of scotch tape on top of it to remind you to keep it curved until you can remember on your own.

2. Dropping your hands to the side is a good way to release accumulated tension.

Use Strong Fingers

One of the problems with the standard keyboard is that all the important keys—such as Shift, Control, Alt, Tab, and Enter—are placed near the weakest finger, the pinkie. Instead of using the little fingers to strike these keys, use a strong, stable finger (such as the index finger) or two fingers (such as the index and middle) to strike these keys. When you use the middle finger, use it *with* the index or ring finger, keeping all the fingers relaxed and curved.

This technique will slow you down a little, but that's not a bad thing. It is better to use a strong finger for a job than stress a weak one.

Exercise for Using Strong Fingers

Position both your right middle and ring fingers over the Shift key. Hold it down and make a capital T using the index finger of your left hand to strike the T.

Use Fingers from Both Hands for Two-Key Strokes

Don't stretch your fingers to reach two keys at once. Many people contort their hands to reach a function key and the Alt key at the same time. Some typists also keep the Shift key down and stretch to reach the letter they are trying to capitalize with the same hand. Don't do this. Use one finger from each hand to strike the keys and keep them in good position while you do.

Use a Light Touch

For some reason, people associate making lots of noise on the keyboard with working hard. Get this idea right out of your head—all it does is make your fingers sore. Pounding on the computer keyboard is the equivalent of dancing on a concrete floor: Both lead to pain and injury. Instead, consciously try to use the lightest possible touch. Think of caressing the keys, not smashing them.

There are also people who press down on the keys until their joints collapse or their fingers blanch, which is another habit to avoid.

Exercise for Using a Light Touch

Type a sample sentence using the lightest touch possible. Type "I always use a light touch when I type."—or another sentence that

---

RULES FOR SAFE COMPUTER USE

1. Maintain neutral wrist positioning.
2. Never rest wrists while typing.
3. Use the whole arm to move hand.
4. Keep fingers curved.
5. Use strong fingers.
6. Use a light touch.
7. Work at a comfortable pace.
8. Take frequent breaks.
9. Keep your fingernails short.
10. Stretch frequently.

will get you in the mood to use good technique or remind you of a habit you are trying to break. Other good samples include "I always keep my wrists straight."; "I remember to take breaks."

Keep Your Fingernails Short

Long fingernails can contribute to RSI. To type with long fingernails, you must use the flat of the finger instead of the fingertip, and to do so requires that you "co-contract" the muscles, that is, hold both the extensor and flexor muscles rigid at the same time. Most people gladly cut their nails if it means being able to use their hands without pain.

TECHNIQUES FOR MOUSE USERS

Using a mouse can be even tougher on the hands than using a keyboard; instead of distributing the work between ten fingers, the burden is placed on one. You also have to keep sliding around to position the icon where you want it, which requires a lot of sustained fine movement and continuous contractions of various small muscles.

Mouse users risk tendinitis of the wrist, deQuervain's disease, and trigger finger. A lot of them get into trouble because they grip the mouse too hard. According to Robert Markison, if you apply ten pounds of pressure gripping an object with the thumb, it puts 100 pounds of pressure on the joint at the base of the thumb, which is ill-equipped to deal with such stress.

If you must use a mouse, the same general principles that apply to desk height and wrist rests also apply here (the click button should be level with the keys of the computer). Talk to an occupational therapist about adapting the shape of the mouse to fit your hand.

How to Handle Your Mouse

1. Mice should be held loosely. Imagine you are holding a small bird. You may not realize it, but gripping creates tension in the other fingers.

2. Don't rest your wrist or forearm on the table while you move the mouse.

3. Use your whole arm and shoulder to move the mouse, not just the wrist.

4. Be careful not to lift your pinkie. Hold the mouse lightly with all of your fingers.

5. Keep your wrist in neutral position.

6. Use a light touch when you click.

HOW TO HANDLE YOUR STYLUS

Penlike styluses present difficulties for the same reason pens do; people hold them too tightly. This is a practice that can lead to trigger finger or writer's cramp. Robert Markison estimates that 25 to 50% of his patients whose injuries are computer-related can't do any handwriting at all; those who are able to write can do it only for an hour or so a day, so a stylus is obviously not a good alternative to a keyboard in this case.

A stylus should be used only on a horizontal surface, not an upright computer screen. Follow steps one and four of the mice rules. Use a pen expander (page 171).

BUILDING ENDURANCE BY PACING YOURSELF

The key to building endurance is pacing. Regaining endurance may require months and sometimes years of careful adherence to the program. You will also need to learn how to pace yourself on the job before you can work safely. You must first determine your "tolerance level"—the amount of time you can work without triggering pain.

How to Determine Your Tolerance Level

To determine how much time you can safely spend at the keyboard, do the following:

1. *Time yourself.* Note the time when you start typing. At the first instant you feel any symptoms (which can be pain, heaviness, or even slight discomfort), stop working and note the amount of time that has passed.

2. *Subtract ten minutes.* Take the time you were able to work without pain and subtract ten minutes. For example, if you work for twenty minutes without pain and subtract ten minutes, that leaves ten minutes. This is your tolerance level. This means you can work for ten minutes and then rest for ten minutes, until your endurance increases. The point is to stop *before* you feel pain; once the pain cycle starts, it is hard to stop. These signals mean the muscles are in distress, and there is evidence that a constant barrage of pain stimuli can result in a chronic pain disorder.

3. *If it hurts, stop.* Don't work for more than thirty minutes at a time without a five- to ten-minute break, and *if you feel pain, stop the pain-causing activity (this could be writing or other nonkeyboard uses of the hand), even if you haven't reached your maximum tolerance time.*

THE HAND SURGEON'S WARM-UP

Robert Markison performs a special hand warm-up every morning. I have adapted it here for RSI.

1. Gently squeeze a sponge in a tepid bubble bath. (Aloe vera is a nice choice.)
2. Using a lotion or oil, massage your fingers and forearms, from fingertip to elbow, paying special attention to the joints.
3. Gently stretch your fingers with the other hand, one by one.
4. Gently stretch your forearms, as illustrated on pages 109–110.
5. Hold your hand to your cheek. Does it feel cold? If so, put on fingerless gloves.

Dr. Markison also keeps his fingers nimble by practicing coin tricks and sleight-of-hand during the day.

THE SENSIBLE BREAK

Here are a few pointers about breaks.

1. Take one 5- to 10-minute break every 25 to 30 minutes at the keyboard. In between, take mini-breaks:
   Rest your hands palm-up on your wrist rest at the end of a paragraph, section, or page for a moment;

   or

   stop and gently turn your head from left to right or *slightly* up and all the way down;

   or

   do some shoulder rolls;

   or

   do nothing for a moment.

2. At least once an hour, take your stretch break. Do a few of the office stretches mentioned in Chapter 11. Overstretching can strain your muscles, so even though you want to get well, remember that moderation is the key. Don't overdo it.

3. Breaks don't imply absolute idleness. If you aren't stretching or icing, you can find something productive to do, such as copying, proofreading, or consulting with coworkers. Be creative. If your boss doesn't understand why you need breaks, get a doctor's note explaining it. (See page 158.)

It is better to stay at an even plateau than to push too hard and have to start building up your endurance all over again after a relapse.

Stopping the activity that causes pain doesn't mean you have to be idle. Find something else to do, such as proofreading, copying, or making a business call.

Warm Up, Cool Down

As you improve, you may gradually increase your keyboard time. Do a few warm-up sets of ten minutes each, with rest breaks. Then do some 12-minute sets. As you wind down your work day, go back to ten-minute "cooldown" sets.

Slow Down

Don't type at top speed constantly, especially if you have to strain to do that. Find a comfortable, steady pace that feels right to you.

Don't Compete

Your total daily keyboard time will be unique to you, so don't expect to keep up with someone else's pace. The key to finding your safe upward limit of daily work time is listening to your body.

Don't Overdo It

It is okay to feel like your hands, shoulders, and forearms have worked out, but you shouldn't be in pain when you go home at night.

Eventually, after timing yourself a lot, you might find that you can pace yourself by "feel" rather than by the clock. Your body will develop a built-in sense of good pacing.

PACING DURING THE CREATIVE PROCESS

Some writers, journalists, and other creative people don't take breaks amid a blaze of inspiration for fear they will lose a good thought or phrase. Years of habit, fear of losing their creativity, or just plain being so immersed in their thoughts that they are unaware of time passing prevents them from adopting safer pacing. If this applies to you, try the technique below. It can also be useful for people who must slow down their speech for voice-activated computers.

Train Memory to Hold Thoughts

Next time you are writing and the timer goes off for a break, stop immediately, even if you're in midsentence. Fix in your mind the thought you were about to write. Tell yourself to remember it the moment you sit down at the keyboard again.

We all get—and forget—wonderful ideas, but learn to trust the creative process. If a great idea came forth once, you can't lose it. Eventually it will resurface, maybe even in better form than it did the first time around.

If you are blocked when you go back to work, try an old writer's trick: Retype the last sentence you wrote. That will usually get you started again.

Unlearn Bad Habits

During one retraining session, a novelist confessed, "You'd die if you could see me at home. I type like this [with her feet on the desk, spine slouched, keyboard in lap]." When she learned that such posture would lead to problems, she said, "But I can't write sitting up. I can't think like that."

I suggested a program where she would be allowed to lounge all she wanted while courting the muse, but she would have to train herself to hold the thought, and then sit up in good position when she typed it. The plan was that eventually she could learn to compose in an upright position without fear of losing creativity.

On further investigation, she confessed that her desk, which was made of a board across two filing cabinets, was too high for comfortable typing, so she held the keyboard on her lap. I suggested she open the drawers of the file cabinets and span the gap with some plywood, which would lower her keyboard to an appropriate height. This solution would cost her $6.00—and may save her career, considering the implications of what she was doing.

The cause of aberrant postures such as lounging, sitting with one foot under your rear end, or leaning on one elbow may be due to a muscle or skeletal imbalance that should be addressed in physical therapy. Tell your doctor and physical therapist the truth about how you sit so they can help you find solutions. It may be as simple as using a footrest for one foot (if you sit with your foot under your hip), exercises to balance the muscles, or some deep tissue massage.

Compose in Your Head

Joseph DePietro, the medical director for the *New York Times*, postulates that one reason older reporters aren't being injured at the rate of their younger colleagues is that they don't rely as heavily on the keyboard. "The old-timers used to write their stories in their heads," said Dr. DePietro. "When they sat down to the typewriter, it would come out perfectly the first time."

CHAPTER 17

Preventing RSI: The Big Picture

The biggest problem in the world could have been solved when it was small.

— Witter Bynner (1881–1968)

With planning and foresight, RSI can be prevented. People who can control pacing and their environment are in the best position to protect themselves. By following the instructions for workstation setup, pacing, and technique retraining outlined in Chapters 15 and 16 faithfully, you should be able to avoid injury. But if you have no control over your pacing, environment, or workstation, things might not be so simple. You will need to negotiate safe working conditions with your employer.

By redesigning jobs, educating the work force about RSI, investing in sound ergonomic equipment, and training employees how to use it, management can head problems off at the pass. A cooperative effort between labor and management such as the one suggested below could solve many of the problems that lead to RSI.

However, if business ignores the contributing factors that lead to RSI, such as machine pacing and improper workstation design, it will pay the hard way: through lost productivity, high insurance, Worker's Compensation, and disability rates and lawsuits. Things are looking up, though: Some companies have come up with innovative approaches to preventing RSI.

℞ FOR RSI

Here, in a nutshell, are some suggestions that labor and management could work on together. Some of these goals cannot be met overnight, of course, but moving in this direction would be worthwhile.

Slow Down

Employees must be allowed to work at their own pace and take breaks. Keyboard workloads must be reduced so that employees aren't overburdened.

This could be accomplished without waste of labor dollars if other non-computer tasks were incorporated in job descriptions.

Stop Splintering and Deskilling Jobs

Instead of splintering and deskilling jobs, enlarge and energize them. "Repetitive tasks are performed best by a machine," wrote Vern Putz-Anderson in *Cumulative Trauma Disorders*. Variety is the spice of life and essential to health. Why expect human beings to do jobs that bore and dispirit them? Jobs should be designed so that workers can fully employ their talents, instead of endlessly repeating the same routine. Rather than watering down tasks, jobs should be made more complicated and challenging—within moderation. Taylorism has outlived its usefulness, and creative systems could replace it.

As Paul Hawken put it in *Growing a Business*, meaningless routine alienates workers. "It is possible for ... the office worker who processes medical insurance claims to work with pride and efficiency, but it's not easy to maintain that attitude. We were not created in order to spend half or more of our waking lives in such constricting circumstances, and we know it."

Hawken makes another good point, too: If you can't give your job your all, it wears you out. Most people, most of the time, Hawken asserts, hold something or even a lot back from their employers because 100 percent of the employee's intelligence, creativity, energy, and abilities is not being utilized and nurtured. "This doesn't mean they are not bone-weary at night; they are, and part of the reason they are is because of this restraint. It's tiring not to put your heart and soul into your work," he declares.

Stay in Shape

Employees who use computers should be encouraged to take responsibility for keeping their bodies strong, supple, and lean. The principles of good upper body conditioning need to be learned—as well as which exercises might be harmful or counterproductive for injured workers. Employers could help by subsidizing memberships in gyms or offering in-house exercise classes, as some smart corporations do already.

Use Sound Design

Workstations, keyboards, and chairs must be designed to fit workers; workers should not be expected to contort their bodies to fit given equipment. Businesses could save millions of dollars spent on expensive consultations about workstation design by asking the real experts: the workers themselves. The person doing the job is often the best judge of flawed workstation setup, and that advice is free.

Start Retraining Programs

All the ergonomic equipment in the world won't prevent RSI unless people who use computer keyboards learn how to type safely, pace themselves, and care for their upper bodies. Safe keyboard techniques should be taught in typing schools, high schools, and job training programs.

Stop Expecting Furniture to Solve Job-Design Problems

According to a survey of 8,000 intensive computer users conducted by the Communications Workers of America, furniture alone won't stop RSI. Said David LeGrande, director of safety and health for CWA, "Since 1989, employers have introduced a lot of new equipment. The majority of respondents say that they have adjustable VDTs, good furniture and keyboards. But physical symptoms have *not* decreased. We've found higher rates of tendinitis and cysts and a whopping 50–100% increase in carpal tunnel syndrome, depending on the occupation. This is indicative of a theory many of us have believed for a long time, which is if you don't look at work organization, you don't solve much." Study jobs as well as workstations: Is there a way to reconstruct them so they aren't so keyboard intensive?

Protect Your Employees

Treat your employees the way you'd like to be treated on the job. Happy employees are productive employees. Workers who don't feel their best can't give their best, and certainly no one can feel enthusiastic about doing work that hurts.

WHEN ALL ELSE FAILS, WORK FOR YOURSELF

Some employees will never be happy in any job because they are entrepreneurs at heart. If you're really unhappy working for others, why not start your own business? When you are your own boss, you can do things your way, but you must also bear the risks and meet the payroll. However, if you are happier as a result, the extra responsibilities would be worth it.

RETHINKING HOW COMPANIES ARE MANAGED

There are some heartening signs of change on the horizon. *Inc. Magazine*, for instance, devoted its cover story to the topic of new innovations in management. It highlighted several companies who have abandoned the techniques of Taylorism, which ultimately created a breeding ground for RSI, in favor of more humane ways of organizing work. With this new approach, employees are let in on decisions that affect them or the company, and through profit sharing and other schemes they are made to feel and think like owners—and profits are up.

Instead of employing the old methods, which divide management and employees into two camps, us and them, everyone works together. "Managers don't have to figure out how to motivate lethargic employees. Workers don't sit around waiting for instructions (and cursing their idiot supervisors in the meantime)." Owners, of course, don't need to be motivated—they know what needs to be done and do it.

According to a report in the *Wall Street Journal*, companies are fighting computer-related tension in various ways described above. Workers at Blue Cross and Blue Shield of Texas are required to stop work and exercise periodically. One software maker in Texas, Micrografx, lets employees work flexible hours and use a company health club during the day. At its San Francisco travel reservation center, American Express trains computer workers to do back-office jobs so they don't spend all day at their computers quoting prices.

Stay Tuned

At this writing, RSI among computer workers is still a new phenomenon. We've brought you the best information available at deadline, but things are changing all the time. Keep informed, because a new breakthrough could be just what you need.

If you have any comments or suggestions for future editions of this book, please write. Sorry, we cannot offer advice on individual problems.

Dr. Emil Pascarelli
Deborah Quilter
The Miller Institute
425 West 59th Street
New York, NY 10019

We have received many requests for videotapes of the exercises and other techniques described in this book. If you want to be notified when they are ready, please send your name, address, and zip code.

PART 5

LEGAL ISSUES

CHAPTER 18

Protecting Your Legal Rights If You Have Job-Related RSI

Most people work for someone else, and even if you are blessed with an understanding and accommodating employer you may need to know your legal rights. Because RSI is so frequently work-related, all kinds of complications come into play that would not affect another sort of injury or disease. Depending on the severity of the injury, these problems can range in magnitude from minor frustration to serious depression brought on by financial chaos or unemployment.

You need to know your rights before you can stand up for them, and it is best to be forewarned rather than caught off guard. If you are injured on the job, do as much research on your rights as you can before you need to exercise them.

Repetitive strain injury has plagued occupations that existed far before the advent of the computer, such as meatpackers and garment industry and assembly line workers. Because doctors, insurers, Workers' Compensation officials, and employers are unfamiliar with computer-related RSI, those who are even temporarily disabled by RSI often face a very tough ordeal. Some people feel too intimidated by the paperwork and pseudolegal proceedings to file claims for money that is rightfully due them under Workers' Compensation. The majority of those who do file must face a hearing at which their claim of injury may be contested. Many people describe the nightmare of having to prove an injury that no one can see. It was a major battle to get carpal tunnel syndrome, for instance, accepted by the Workers' Compensation Board in New York state. The hearing process can frighten and frustrate people who need physical therapy or other treatment—but can't get it until their claim is approved by the Workers' Compensation Board or insurance carrier. This may change as the level of awareness about RSI grows, but for the moment, it makes things even harder for the patients.

WORKERS' COMPENSATION

Workers' Compensation was designed to allow people who are injured on the job to be paid regardless of whose fault it was; however, the amount of damages they can recover are limited. So there is a trade-off: Workers' Compensation prevents employees from suing their employers and also limits the amount of damages people can receive.

Workers' Compensation rules change from state to state. You might need help figuring them out: You could call your local Workers' Compensation office, or find an attorney who specializes in this area of law. (See the Resources section, page 208.)

Problems with Workers' Compensation

Lower than Usual Fees. If Workers' Compensation paid the doctors' and therapists' usual fee, maybe people wouldn't be so angry with it. Because Workers' Compensation pays according to its own schedule, many doctors and therapists refuse to accept Workers' Compensation patients.

Stigma. Workers' Compensation patients are often stigmatized as being uncooperative malingerers by the medical profession. Though a few people try to take advantage of the system, it is certainly not the rule. Said Dr. Joseph DePietro, medical director of the *New York Times,* "I have seen a lot of phonies in my career, but to compare this type of claim with RSI is absolutely insane. I have trouble getting people to *rest.*"

Uncooperative Doctors. Many RSI patients' doctors refuse to attribute their injury to their job when it is indeed the source of their injury, thus disallowing their Workers' Compensation claim. Two separate problems are possible here: The doctor either is uninformed about RSI or doesn't want to accept Workers' Compensation cases because of the nuisance. So Workers' Compensation patients often must scramble to find a doctor who will take care of them.

Long Waits. Sometimes patients who are frightened and hurting must wait months for their claim to be approved before beginning physical therapy, when it is critical to stop the cycle of pain and injury. Waits of as long as six months for a hearing date are not unusual. Delays in Workers' Compensation payments frustrate the medical staff. Even after a claim is accepted, patients can face stiff obstacles in the effort to get treatment. Sometimes they must get a lawyer and have a hearing just to continue physical therapy.

Delays in treatment can have dire consequences: If reflex sympathetic dysfunction, a serious nerve disorder that sometimes results from RSI, is not treated in time, it can mean a life of chronic excruciating pain. At present, treatment is often delayed while bureaucrats argue about who pays for what.

Lots of Red Tape. Patients aren't the only ones who become frustrated with the bureaucratic red tape involved with Workers' Compensation claims. Doctors, office personnel, and rehabilitation therapists all bemoan the paperwork and annoyance it causes. It is not unusual for a doctor to spend two hours per patient on paperwork during the course of treatment. "This does not include paperwork documenting disability for state or federal disability applications which are sometimes filed by patients whose symptoms are the most severe and cannot return to employment in their profession," noted George Piligian, a doctor who treats RSI patients at the Miller Institute.

"One of my big gripes against Workers' Comp is that it will gladly shell out $3,000 for a carpal tunnel release without even asking questions, but when I do a year of psychotherapy, I have to justify it—and psychotherapy probably helps them more," added Robert Rosenthal, a psychiatrist who specializes in helping patients cope with RSI or chronic pain.

Subtle Harassment. To add to the patients' worries, some employers—and insurers—fail to understand that an injury years in the making doesn't bounce back overnight. One man with severe epicondylitis complained that his employer kept calling him to ask when he was coming back. "I cannot *drive* right now. They refuse to understand," he said with disgust. Another woman who could not even shampoo her hair without great effort was being hounded by her insurer's "rehabilitation counselor." "She wants to get me back to work so they don't have to pay me. Her whole job is to harass people so they'll go back to work," she complained.

Vincent Rossillo, a Manhattan attorney who represents a large number of RSI claimants, said the insurance carriers often hire rehabilitation nurses to subtly harass you back to work. "They'll come to your home and they'll go to your doctor's appointments with you and sit with you and explain things. At first they're very nice, but then they start questioning the doctor, and they ask him if you could come back to work. And the doctor might finally say, 'She could *try* going back to work,' and the next thing you know, they write to the carrier and say the patient can go back to work so they can reduce the benefits."

Insurers, of course, must protect themselves from a minority of people who attempt to defraud the Workers' Compensation system, usually with ailments that are not visible, such as headache, backache, or neck pain. So some insurance carriers send an investigator to your house to ask for information about your health that can be used against you later in a hearing. The investigators might even question your neighbors about you. Unsuspecting people tend to answer the questions because the investigators look official, but Rossillo said he advised against answering their questions. "I would advise people not to cooperate," Rossillo said.

It may seem innocent for an investigator to ask about your hobbies, but if you mention that you knit or play a musical instrument, the insurance carrier may try to attribute your RSI to that rather than to the long hours of computer work you do.

Who Is Eligible for Workers' Compensation

If you are employed, you are most likely covered by Workers' Compensation. Independent contractors or self-employed people are not covered unless they carry their own policy. Your injury must arise out of your employment, and there must be a medical basis for your claim.

When to File

You should file your claim as soon as you are injured. In New York State, for instance, you have two years from the day you knew, or should have known, that your condition is work-related to file a claim. "People shouldn't let their doctor or anyone else talk them out of it," he advised. "They should seek a doctor who is familiar with these occupational conditions, and if the doctor thinks it is work-related, they should file—no matter what their employer or anyone else would say."

There is no penalty for filing for Workers' Compensation, according to Rossillo. If you fail to receive it, the claim would simply be disallowed. Be sure not to confuse *notifying* your employer with *filing* a claim. Rules change from state to state, so if there is any doubt, call your Workers' Compensation board to see if they have a record of your claim.

The Hearing

People usually dread facing Workers' Compensation hearings, where they must prove something is wrong with them to a hearing officer or they won't get their benefits. They say they are made to feel like criminals, demeaned or unappreciated. Ironically, the people who develop RSI are usually the hardest workers.

At the hearings, the insurance carrier's representative advises the judge of its position, and the judge reviews the medical evidence to see if it meets the requirements. Claimants may be examined by an insurance company doctor. If the insurance company still denies the claim, the claimant and a witness from the company will testify about the type of work the claimant does; if the claim is still controverted after that, the doctors for both sides will testify.

The judge will make a ruling, which either side may appeal. If the insurance company loses, it generally files an appeal. It doesn't have to pay the award if the case is on appeal.

Deciding Whether You Need an Attorney

If your Workers' Compensation claim is contested, you may need an attorney. Technically, you don't have to have one, but according to Rossillo, "The insurance company always has a representative there, and his job is to pay as little as possible in these cases, so I would certainly recommend it." One woman said she was very relieved to have an attorney by her side during her hearing; he also explained some legalese that she feared meant her claim might be denied but was actually just intimidating language for a routine procedure.

There may be drawbacks to having an attorney handle your case, however. John Burton, director of the Institute of Management and Labor Relations at Rutgers University, conducted a study comparing the total amounts of benefits for claimants who used lawyers with the benefits for those who didn't. He found that when lawyers are involved in settling lump-sum payments, the amount of the benefits is lower, at least in New York state. Dr. Burton noted that in some states, the only way attorneys get decent fees from the Workers' Compensation system is through lump-sum payments. But if you accept lump-sum payments, you are for all practical purposes no longer eligible for further benefits, he added. "Workers ought to recognize that accepting settlements rather than weekly, ongoing payments may not be in their best interest," he warned.

Finding an Attorney

Use the same technique to find an attorney that you use to find a doctor, accountant, or any other consultant. Get names from friends or associates, talk to two or three, and see who strikes you as the best. Your attorney should be accessible and speak in a way you understand.

Workers' Compensation is a very specialized area of law, and there are attorneys who limit their practice to Workers' Compensation cases, so try to find one of those if you can. There may be a Workers' Compensation bar association in your state. Licensed representatives will also appear on behalf of claimants at hearings in some states. See page 208 for more information on getting legal help.

Fees

Workers' Compensation cases are paid on a contingency basis. The Workers' Compensation Board sets the fee depending on the services that were rendered on behalf of the person and amount of the award. As a matter of general practice, it is a good idea to let doctors and lawyers wait for Workers' Compensation to reimburse them.

NOTE: In some states, it is against the law for a licensed representative or an attorney to accept money from a claimant directly, and if there isn't any award made, there is no fee. It is also illegal for a doctor to accept payment directly from a patient in a Workers' Compensation claim in some states.

THE AMERICANS WITH DISABILITIES ACT

The Americans with Disabilities Act (ADA) was instituted in 1992 to protect the rights of people with disabilities. At present, the law applies only to companies with 25 or more employees. Employers with 15 or more employees will be covered beginning July 26, 1994.

Under the ADA, the term *disability* is described as a "physical or mental impairment that substantially limits one or more major life activities." This could apply to RSI because performing manual tasks, a major life activity under the ADA, requires the ability to use your hands in normal fashion.

If you have a disability, your employer is required to provide a "reasonable accommodation" for you to do your job. Reasonable accommodation could mean a number of things, such as a change in scheduling, providing for breaks, or offering a different job if another one is available. However, the ADA does not require employers to reduce their quality or production standards, so if you produce only 70% of your previous level, for example, the employer would not be required to keep you. An employer may reassign you to "light duty" or another position if it can't accommodate your current job, but it is not required to create a new job for you.

The ADA is not specific about implementation, because it anticipates that employer and employee will try to find solutions together. Because disabilities and the nature of work can vary drastically, each request for reasonable accommodation must be made on a case-by-case basis. If you think you need a new chair to perform your work adequately, for instance, it may or may not be covered. The ADA does not require employers to make accommodations that would place an "undue hardship" on their business. So if you work for a large corporation, the outlay of several hundred dollars for a new chair may not be considered an undue hardship, but if you work for a small company, it may.

Under the ADA, you can sue your employer, not for the injury, but for discrimination if they do not provide reasonable accommodation for you. Jobseekers should be aware that prospective employers are not allowed to ask medical questions during a hiring interview, so you may also sue if you feel you were not hired for a job you were qualified to do. Other remedies include reinstatement, back pay, and court orders to stop discrimination.

Because the law is so new, many questions about how it applies to RSI are yet to be decided by the courts. However, if you think that your employer has discriminated against you, contact the Equal Employment Opportunity Commission. (See the Resources section.)

LAWSUITS

Employees cannot sue their employers for injuries because of Workers' Compensation laws, so many people are opting to sue the manufacturers under product liability laws, claiming that the manufacturers should have known their products would cause injuries. In a lawsuit against 96 keyboard manufacturers that consolidates nearly 400 claims in the United States District Court for the Eastern District of New York, plaintiffs are seeking compensatory damages for lost income, present and future medical expenses related to RSI, impairment of their future earning capacity, and pain and suffering. In addition, they seek punitive damages, which could be awarded if the jury finds the manufacturers guilty of willful and wanton conduct by failure to warn people about the hazards of their keyboards. There are also derivative suits on behalf of spouses who now must take over duties formerly performed by their injured mate. No one is sure how the courts will eventually rule on these cases, but they are being watched with great interest.

THE MYTH OF PRIVACY

People understandably wonder whether they will be fired if they have permanent partial disability, or whether they will be employable again. There are no simple answers to these questions. You should know, however, that some employers might use data banks to screen job applicants who file for Workers' Compensation. According to *Privacy for Sale* by Jeffrey Rothfeder, Employers Information Service, Inc. (EIS), a Louisiana data bank, maintains more than a million files on workers primarily in the Gulf Coast area in oil, gas, construction, and other heavy industries who apply for Workers' Compensation and those who sue their employers after an accident. "What EIS knows is important to these employers because workmen's compensation are overwhelming businesses . . . EIS stresses that its purpose is simply to provide objective information, and not to make it impossible for workmen's compensation claimants to find work."

Not only that, getting health insurance may be problematic: Rothfeder also mentions the Medical Information Bureau (MIB), whose data banks contain summaries of health conditions on more than 15 million Americans and Canadians. MIB, a nonprofit association comprising 750 life insurance companies, was formed to prevent insurance fraud among policyholders. "Insurance companies feed MIB's cavernous mainframes whatever they learn about individuals from insurance applications, physicians' files, and hospital records," writes Rothfeder. Then, when someone applies for a policy, underwriters scan MIB's computers to see whether the applicant has an existing data file. Neil Day, the president of MIB, refused to say whether or not RSI was among the health conditions listed in MIB's codes.

According to Harvie Raymond, Director of Insurance Products for the Health Insurance Association of America, in most cases new hires are covered by health insurers with no questions asked. However, if someone with a history of RSI applied for private health or disability insurance, there are four possible outcomes: The coverage would be granted as requested; the carrier would issue a policy with a waiver that claims would be covered except for RSI for a certain period of time; it would offer coverage for an additional premium; or the carrier would decline to insure the person. "Some carriers use MIB for health insurance; some do not," said Raymond. "I would expect disability insurers would check with MIB." If someone does not mention having a medical condition that has bearing on the decision to issue a policy, the policy could be canceled by the carrier.

FOR THE PERMANENTLY/PARTIALLY DISABLED

RSI is no joke. Just because you don't see an open wound doesn't mean a person is not seriously injured. Some people can be totally disabled, not just for months, but for years or their entire lives. Even classifying what exactly constitutes disability is difficult. Here is an example: A woman might have trouble picking up her child because it causes intense pain. But another woman fears that if her four-year-old boy ran in front of a car, she wouldn't be able to restrain him. One disability causes inconvenience; the other could be life threatening. There are too many degrees of impairment within this disease to make hard-and-fast statements.

With RSI, nobody really knows what the long-term outlook is. For the moment, people who pass the point of no return can't be helped physically, but there are a number of other things they can do to better their lives.

OSHA AND STATE LEGISLATION

The Occupational Safety and Health Administration (OSHA) is studying RSI, but it has not developed final rules in this regard. According to a report in the *New York Times*, an administrative law judge dismissed a $1.3 million fine OSHA had imposed on Pepperidge Farms for willfully disregarding the repetitive stress problems of 69 of 175 nonunion bakery workers. The judge threw out the fine "because there is no Federal standard dealing with repetitive stress."

UNION INVOLVEMENT

Because RSI is a job-related injury, unions are very concerned about it. Communications Workers of America (CWA), for instance, has pressured NIOSH and OSHA to research RSI and allowed its members to be studied. CWA has also pushed for protective regulations and laws; it does collective bargaining for people who work for telephone companies and local municipalities; it educates its members about their rights; and it helps them get good medical care.

Joel Shufro, executive director of the New York Committee for Occupational Safety and Health, said that his group, which is a nonprofit coalition of local unions and activists, is attempting to get the New York state legislature to fund a program that would pay for people's immediate medical needs if their employers' Workers' Compensation insurance carriers contest their claim for RSI. Such measures could mean the difference between permanent serious disability and being able to reverse the course of the injury.

The unions are also very concerned about the way video display terminals are handled in contracts. Some unions have insisted on free annual eye examinations for their members, for instance.

DISABILITY BENEFITS

Disability benefits under Workers' Compensation fall into several categories: temporary disability, temporary total disability, permanent total disability, temporary partial disability, and permanent partial disability. The amount of money you receive is based on a percentage of your weekly wages, with an upward limit. For most people, there are no cost-of-living increases.

Vocational Rehabilitation

All states offer vocational and educational services for people with disabilities. In New York state, for instance, the office of Vocational and Educational Services for Individuals with Disabilities (VESID) will provide vocational and career counseling; job training, including college, university, trade and business school programs; books, tools, and equipment you may need for training or employment; some costs of modifying equipment at work or home; job placement; counseling; and many other services. There is no cost for meeting with a VESID counselor, but there are eligibility criteria: You must be disabled, and there must be a reasonable chance that you could become employed if you receive their services. You also may be required to pay for some services based on your income or family resources. See the Resources section for more information on rehabilitation services.

Things You Should Know

- It is common for employers to controvert claims for RSI. Don't assume that you will lose your benefits if this happens.
- Some unions and other organizations have workshops where you can get free advice.
- Many people are not aware that psychotherapy may be covered under Workers' Comp.
- It is legal for a potential employer to inquire about your Workers' Compensation history *after* a conditional job offer has been made, not before.
- An employer may make you a job offer on the condition that you have a medical examination if this is required of all potential employees in the same job category. The post-offer examination may not disqualify a disabled person who can currently perform essential job functions on the basis of the possibility of future injuries. Information from such medical inquiries must be filed separately from personnel records and be kept confidential.
- If you knowingly provide a false answer about your health to an employer in a legal question after you have been offered a job, you may be fired, or not hired.
- Information from medical inquiries may not be used to discriminate against the employee.
- Filing a third-party lawsuit against a keyboard manufacturer, or even an ADA-based suit, may also make it hard for you to find another job.

Reference Notes

Chapter 1

1. **Ramazzini** Hunter J. H. Fry, "The Effect of Overuse on the Musician's Technique: A Comparative and Historical Review," *International Journal of Arts Medicine* 1(1) (Fall 1991):46.

3. **a cover story in *Information Week*** Doug Bartholomew, "Repetitive Strain Injuries cost business $20 billion a year—Is it your problem?" *Information Week,* 9 Nov. 1992, 33.

4. **Stewart B. Leavitt** Stewart B. Leavitt "The Healthy Office of the '90s" (paper funded by HAG, Inc., 1992), 2.

6. **In her book *In the Age*** Shoshana Zuboff, *In the Age of the Smart Machine: The Future of Work and Power* (New York: Basic Books, 1988), 315–61.

6. **the authors of *Healthy Work*** Robert Karasek and Töres Theorell, *Healthy Work: Stress, Productivity, and the Reconstruction of Working Life* (New York: Basic Books, 1990), 262.

6. **In his book *Technostress*** Craig Brod, *Technostress: The Human Cost of the Computer Revolution* (Reading, MA: Addison-Wesley, 1984), 45.

11. **An Australian study of an RSI epidemic** Yolande Lucire, "Neurosis in the workplace," *Medical Journal of Australia* 145 (6 Oct. 1986), 325.

11. **another Australian study** Wayne Hall and Louise Morrow, "Repetition Strain Injury: An Australian Epidemic of Upper Limb Pain," *Social Science Medicine* 27, 67(1988):646.

Chapter 2

13. **Common sense is** Charles Robert Lightfoot, comp., *Handbook of Business Quotations: Choice Words of Business Wisdom for Successful Speeches, Reports, Letters, and Papers* (Houston, Tex.: Gulf Publishing Company, 1991), 36.

Chapter 4

36. **Hans Selye, whose book** Hans Selye, *The Stress of Life,* rev. ed. (New York: McGraw-Hill Book Co., 1956, 1976, 1978), 1.

37. **In the book *Healthy Work*** Robert Karasek and Töres Theorell, *Healthy Work: Stress, Productivity, and the Reconstruction of Working Life* (New York: Basic Books, 1990), 16, 108.

38. **You live badly** Quoted in Alfred Kazin, "The Way We Live Now," review of *Culture of Complaint: The Fraying of Ameria,* by Robert Hughes, *The New York Review of Books,* 22 April 1993.

38. **"Americans continue to get fatter,"** "Americans Found Retreating From Healthy Eating Habits," *New York Times,* 14 March 1993.

39. **as Hooshang Hooshmand points out** Hooshang Hooshmand, *Chronic Pain: Reflex Sympathetic Dysfunction Prevention and Management* (Boca Raton, Fla.: CRC Press, 1993), 97–98, 116.

40. **Nearly three out of five** Jane Brody, "Unkindest Cut: Children's Fitness," *New York Times,* 3 Feb. 1993.

Chapter 6

50. **According to the National Institute** Thomas Hales, Steven Sauter, Marty Petersen, Vern Putz-Anderson, Laurence Fine, Troy Ochs, Larry Schleifer, and Bruce Bernard, "Health Hazard Evaluation Report, HETA 89-299-2230, US West Communications," National Institute for Occupational Safety and Health, July 1992.

54. **According to Vern Putz-Anderson** Vern Putz-Anderson, ed., *Cumulative Trauma Disorders: A Manual for Musculoskeletal Diseases of the Upper Limbs* (Philadelphia, Penn.: Taylor & Francis, 1988), 17.

59. **Focal dystonia was described** In Hunter J. H. Fry, "The Effect of Overuse on the Musician's Technique: A Comparative and Historical Review," *International Journal of Arts Medicine* 1(1) (Fall 1991): 46–47.

59. **In 1888, W. R. Gowers** W. R. Gowers, *A Manual of Diseases of the Nervous System* (Philadelphia: P. Blakiston, Son & Co., 1888), 1064.

Chapter 7

68. **In my study of injured** Emil Pascarelli and John Jake Kella, "Soft-Tissue Injuries Related to Use of the Computer Keyboard: A Clinical Study of 53 Injured Persons," *Journal of Occupational Medicine* 35, no. 5 (May 1993): 524.

Chapter 8

76. **According to the *United States Pharmacopeia*** *United States Pharmacopeia Complete Drug Reference,* 1993 ed. (Yonkers, N.Y.: Consumer Report Books, 1993).

77. **During a lecture on RSI** From a Harvard Club address given by Robert Markinson, 15 Jan. 1993.

79. **A study published in the *New England Journal*** David M. Eisenberg, Ronald C. Kessler, Cindy Foster, Frances E. Norlock, David R. Calkins, and Thomas L. Delbanco, "Unconventional Medicine in the United States: Prevalence, Costs, and Patterns of Use," *New England Journal of Medicine* 328 (28 Jan. 1993): 246.

80. **A useful analogy** In P. J. Skerrett, "Mighty Vitamins," *Medical World News,* Jan. 1993, 32.

81. **According to a report in the *New York Times*** Jane Brody, "Vitamins as Muscle-Damage Fighter," *New York Times,* 21 Oct. 1992.

Chapter 9

83. **James Sheedy** In "State of the Office," *VDT News,* Jan./Feb. 1992.

84. **It is possible to "charley horse" the eyes** Melvin Schrier, "Eyeing Tax Season," *Practicing CPA,* Dec. 1987, 3.

85. **According to Melvin Schrier** Melvin Schrier, "Eye Problems May Be Cause of CRT User Productivity Limits," *Contract,* March 1983, 103.

85. **Schrier says that your doctor should also test for *hyperphoria*** Melvin Schrier, "Eyeing Tax Season," *Practicing CPA,* Dec. 1987, 3.

Chapter 10

88. **The word *doctor*** Eric Partrige, *Origins: A Short Etymological Dictionary of Modern English* New York: Macmillan, 1958), 161.

91. **"The problem with RSI** From an interview with Jane Bear-Lehman, 3 April 1993.

Chapter 12

121. **I finally convinced my landlord** Quoted in *The RSI Network* newsletter, Issue 10, Feb. 1993.

123. **"Everybody's got a list** From an interview with Jane Bear-Lehman, 3 April 1993.

Chapter 13

133. **All pain is in your head.** From an interview with Dr. Robert Rosenthal, 26 March 1993.

134. **"Part of the problem** From an interview with Dr. Robert Rosenthal, 26 March 1993.

140. **My boss came back** "The Stress of the Job," *Legal Business Magazine*, Jan. Feb. 1992, 9.

144. **If we all could clap** Kathleen Sullivan, "Lending Each Other a Hand," *San Francisco Examiner*, 21 March 1993.

Chapter 15

159. **"When employers make** From a lecture by Charley Richardson, at the Repetitive Strain Injury Conference, North Haven, Conn., March 24, 1993.

162. **What you see on your screen** James E. Sheedy, O.D., PhD, *Eyecare Technology* 3(1)(1993): 34.

Chapter 17

188. **"Repetitive tasks are performed** Vern Putz-Anderson, ed., *Cumulative Trauma Disorders: A Manual for Musculoskeletal Diseases of the Upper Limbs* (Philadelphia, Penn.: Taylor & Francis, 1988), 88.

188. **As Paul Hawken put it** Paul Hawken, *Growing a Business* (New York: Simon & Schuster, 1988), 13, 113–14.

189. **According to a survey** *VDT News*, Jan./Feb. 1992, Editors' Notebook.

189. ***Inc. Magazine*** John Case, "A Company of Businesspeople," *Inc. Magazine,* April 1993, 80.

190. **a report in the *Wall Street Journal*** Christopher Conte, "Fighting Technostress: Exercise and Variety Ease Computer-Related Tension," *Wall Street Journal,* 4 May 1993.

Chapter 18

197. **According to *Privacy for Sale*** Jeffrey Rothfeder, *Privacy for Sale: How Computerization Has Made Everyone's Private Life an Open Secret* (New York: Simon & Schuster, 1992), 154–56, 184.

199. **a report in the *New York Times*** Michael deCourcy Hinds, "Judge Rejects U.S. Penalty for Repetitive Stress Injuries," *New York Times,* 27 March 1993.

Other References (Partial List)

Benjamin, Ben E., with Borden, Gale. *Listen to Your Pain.* New York: Penguin Books, 1984.

Bingham, Beverly. *Cooking with Fragile Hands.* Naples, Fla. Creative Cuisine, Inc., 1985. Out of print.

Cyriax, James. *Textbook of Orthopaedic Medicine.* 8th ed. Vol. 1, *Diagnosis of Soft Tissue Lesions.* London: Baillière Tindall, 1991.

Equal Employment Opportunity Commission. *A Technical Assistance Manual on the Employment Provisions (Title I) of the Americans with Disabilities Act,* January 1992. Available from Superintendent of Documents, P.O. Box 371954, Pittsburgh, PA 15250-7954 for $25.00.

Kasdan, Morton L., ed. *Occupational Hand & Upper Extremity Injuries & Diseases.* Philadelphia, Penn.: Hanley & Belfus, Inc., 1991.

Lister, Graham. *The Hand: Diagnosis and Indications.* 2d ed. Edinburgh: Churchill Livingstone, 1984.

Pećina, Marko M., Krmpotić-Nemanić, Jelena, and Markiewitz, Andrew D. *Tunnel Syndromes*. Boca Raton, Fla.: CRC Press, 1991.

Tubiana, Raoul, ed. *The Hand*. Vol. 4. Philadelphia, Penn.: W. B. Saunders Company, Harcourt Brace Jovanovich, Inc., 1991.

Resources

We have no financial interest in the resources listed below, nor are we necessarily endorsing them. They are provided as a convenience for you. This list is not all-inclusive. Many other sources of help may be available, and you should seek them out. Prices were current at deadline but could have changed.

SUPPORT GROUPS

There may be many more groups than we've listed here. Your doctor or therapist may know of some in your area. If not, see Chapter 13 for ideas about forming your own.

California

East Bay RSI Support Group
Contact: Joan Lichterman
(510) 653-1802

RSI Support Group of San Francisco
Contact: Judy Doane
(415) 931-8780

Santa Rosa RSI Group
Contact: Stephanie Barnes
(707) 571-0397

Marin RSI Support Group
Contact: Liza Smith
(415) 459-0510

SF Peninsula RSI Support Group
Caremark Peninsula Athlete's Center
216 Mosswood Way
So. San Francisco, CA 94080
Contact: Lynda Jensen
(415) 589-0600

Lynda Jensen has prepared a step-by-step blueprint on forming RSI groups that she will share if you write or call her.

Connecticut

The Connecticut Chronic Pain Outreach
Network, Inc.
P.O. Box 388
Hartford, CT 06141-0388

Mutual self-help group offers support, encouragement, and help for those in chronic pain. Write for list of meetings.

New York

RSI Support Group
Mount Sinai–Irving J. Selikoff
   Occupational Health Clinical Center
P.O. Box 1252
One Gustave L. Levy Place
New York, NY 10029-6574
Contact: Susan Nobel, M.S.W.
(212) 241-1527

NEWSLETTERS

Some of these newsletters are aimed at people who need current information about RSI, not the sufferers themselves. Write for a sample before subscribing—if possible—to find out if they are right for you. There are also some excellent newsletters produced by RSI support groups.

The RSI Network

To subscribe, contact Craig O'Donnell:
dadadata@world.std.com at Internet or
   72511,240 at CompuServe
To contribute information or donations:
Caroline Rose, Editor
970 Paradise Way
Palo Alto, CA 94306

This online newsletter with help and news for people with RSI is available on Ziffnet/Mac and CompuServe.

VDT News

P.O. Box 1799 Grand Central Station
New York, NY 10163
$127.00/year (six bimonthly issues). Send a self-addressed 9 × 12 envelope for a sample copy.

This newsletter is for people responsible for computer health and safety, union officials, lawyers, and others interested in computer-related health risks including RSI; office ergonomics; labor-management issues; litigation; and federal, state, and local legislation. VDT News has a special interest in electromagnetic fields.

The Healthy Office Report

Courthouse Place
54 W. Hubbard Street
Suite 403
Chicago, IL 60610

Targeted to clerical professions. Covers sick building syndrome, sexual harassment, and RSI. $35.00/year (12 issues).

Workplace Safety & Health

Courthouse Place
54 W. Hubbard Street
Suite 403
Chicago, IL 60610

This publication deals with federal initiatives, OSHA proclamations, national legislation, and corporate practices relating to workplace health and safety. $35.00/year (12 issues).

CTD News

10 Railroad Ave.
P.O. Box 239
Haverford, PA 19041-0239

This newsletter helps business cope with cumulative trauma disorder. Covers prevention, ergonomics and Workers' Compensation. $125.00/year (10 issues).

Repetitive Stress Injury Litigation Reporter

1646 West Chester Pike
P.O. Box 1000
Westtown, PA 19395
(800) 345-1101

This publication covers rulings on RSI lawsuits all over the country. Court documents are available. $550/year (12 issues) or $325/6 months (6 issues).

GOVERNMENT AGENCIES AND PROGRAMS

U.S. Equal Employment Opportunity Commission

1801 L Street, N.W.
Washington, DC 20507
ADA Helpline (800) 669-EEOC (voice)
or (800) 800-3302 (TDD)

This commission enforces Title I provisions prohibiting discrimination in employment against qualified individuals with disabilities. Provides information, speakers, technical assistance, training, and referral to specialized resources for employers and people with disabilities through headquarters and district offices. Booklets and fact sheets are available.

National Institute of Occupational Safety and Health (NIOSH)

Technical Information Center
4676 Columbia Parkway
Cincinnati, OH 45226
(800) 35NIOSH
FAX: (513) 533-8573

This research group does free literature searches and provides free information packages on a large variety of work-related issues, including chemical hazards and cumulative trauma disorders.

Centers for Independent Living Program

Rehabilitation Services Administration
U.S. Department of Education
Mary E. Switzer Building
330 C St. S.W.
Washington, DC 20202

This program offers services and programs to enable severely disabled people to live independently, including counseling and advocacy services on income benefits and legal rights, loans, personal care assistants, advice on job modifications, and accommodations and assistive devices. Offers recruitment, job training, and job placement services.

Client Assistance Program (CAP)

Mary E. Switzer Building
330 C St. S.W.
Washington, DC 20202
(202) 732-1406 (voice)
or (202) 732-2848 (TDD)

Programs in each state investigate, negotiate, and mediate solutions to problems under the Rehabilitation Act of 1973. CAP provides legal counsel and litigation services to persons unable to obtain adequate legal services.

Job Accommodation Network (JAN)

P.O. Box 6123
809 Allen Hall
Morgantown, WV 26506-6123
(800) 526-7234 or (800) ADA-WORK

The network provides free consulting with professional human factors counselors about custom job and worksite accommodation.

NONGOVERNMENTAL ORGANIZATIONS

For Problems with Workers' Compensation:

Check with your local bar association. Ask if there is a bar association specializing in Workers' Compensation law in your state. Also ask your union for help, if you belong to one.

American Bar Association

Commission on Mental and Physical
  Disability Law
1800 M St., N.W.
Washington, DC 20036
(202) 331-2240

The American Bar Association provides information and technical assistance on all aspects of disability law. It offers training to employers and individuals with disabilities on the Americans with Disabilities Act. It publishes the *Mental and Physical Disability Law Reporter*.

9 to 5: National Association of Working Women

614 Superior Ave., N.W.
Cleveland, OH 44113
(216) 566-9308 or (800) 522-0925
  (job problems hotline)

This association offers information on job rights and legal counseling. Men can join, too. Membership $25.00/year.

FOR OTHER HELP

Carpal Tunnel Syndrome/RSI Association

P.O. Box 514
Santa Rose, CA 95402
Contact: Stephanie Barnes

The Carpal Tunnel Syndrome/RSI Association acts as a clearinghouse for information about RSI, publishes a newsletter, and keeps a list of RSI groups around the country.

American Occupational Therapy Association

1383 Piccard Dr.
P.O. Box 1725
Rockville, MD 20849-1725
(301) 948-9626

This association refers employers and individuals with disabilities to occupational therapists for help with performing job analyses, identifying job accommodations, and modifications. It has local chapters.

TALKING BOOKS

Recording for the Blind

20 Roszel Road
Princeton, NJ 08540
(609) 452-0606 or (800) 221-4792
  (book orders and inquiries)

This nonprofit service provides educational and professional books on audiocassettes to people who have a documented disability that could impair reading. Lifetime membership costs $37.50. Special equipment is required. (*Note:* Recorded books are also available from most public libraries.)

CATALOGS

After Therapy Catalog

(800) 634-4351

Call for free catalog.

Adaptability: Products for Independent Living

(800) 243-9232

Call for free catalog.

Enrichments

(800) 323-5547   Call for free catalog.

These catalogs sell gadgets and gizmos that will help you get through the activities of daily life, from a button-hooker to help you dress in the morning to a Plexiglas® bookholder that suspends over your head so you can read that mystery before you go to sleep. Other useful items are paring boards, graters, and mixing bowls designed to be used with one hand; tools to help you open car doors, use keys, and turn lamp knobs; ergonomic cutlery and pens; and handles for adapting hard-to-operate push buttons. These catalogs offer money-back guarantees on most items.

NOTE: Some of the ergonomic equipment sold by these catalogs and vendors is helpful, but some is of dubious value, so choose wisely.

Index